Life with MIL

A Candid Journey of Alzheimer's
With My Mother-in-law

LISA DAVENPORT

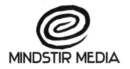

MINDSTIR MEDIA

Published by Mindstir Media, LLC
45 Lafayette Rd | Suite 181| North Hampton, NH 03862 | USA
1.800.767.0531 | www.mindstirmedia.com

Printed in the United States of America
ISBN-13: 978-1-958729-07-6 (paperback)

Dedication

———————

To Joe
My husband, my best friend, my Prince, my forever cheerleader and rock.
I couldn't imagine this ride we call Life without you.

To Ashley & Joey
My beautiful children thank you for all the "grandma sitting."
For the understanding of missed vacations, disrupted dinners, and most of all,
thank you for sharing your parents unconditionally for eight years.

To MIL
My beloved mother-in-law, Rosemary.
A promise is a promise, this is my final gift to you…

Acknowledgments

I want to thank my own mom for her lessons of love, courage, and tolerance. She was instrumental in establishing the strong foundation I needed to build a sturdy structure of love and understanding necessary for life. That foundation was put to the ultimate test on this journey—she prepared me well.

Lisa Lelas and Cindi Dale Pietrzyk, wildly accomplished writers and editors in their own rights, offered their advice and guidance. Cindi, your push early on gave this dyslexic a big confidence boost. Lisa, thanks doesn't seem like enough. I still maintain you were 50 percent therapist and 50 percent writing coach during our monthly meetings. Reliving much of this book was challenging, somehow you made it bearable. Thank you for helping me keep my promise.

I will be forever grateful for the care and unwavering support, patience, and love the staff of Regency House in Wallingford, Connecticut showed not only to Mom, but also to us.

Contents

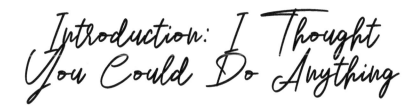

Introduction: I Thought You Could Do Anything

Connecticut

So how did *Life with MIL* come to be? The story was thirty-one years in the making. It was a relationship that defied the odds; daughters-in-law and mothers-in-law aren't "supposed" to be close, they're "supposed" to be rivals. Ours, however, is a story of friendship, respect, and unwavering love; it's a story that needs to be told.

This part of our story begins in 2011. During the last few months of that year, Joe and I had noticed Mom forgetting things here and there. I witnessed a close call while she was driving with our son Joey in the car, a careless mistake that could have been so much worse. She also admitted to getting lost in an adjoining town and losing track of simple conversations. After quite a few doctors' visits and more unsettling events, we knew we would have to do something soon. We had to face the worrisome fact that Mom was slowly slipping away from us. So, on a bright spring afternoon, the kind of day where you pause to appreciate the tulips popping open after a long cold winter, Joe and I were handed a pamphlet about a new research study for Alzheimer's at Yale, we decided to bring the idea up to Mom.

After some convincing, many tears, a lot of anger, and so much love, Mom agreed. I framed the entire process as a "new adventure" for her and I. "It'll be fun," I said. "We'll get to spend lots of time together," I argued. While she may have been skeptical, she was willing. I felt a glimmer of hope. I knew Alzheimer's didn't have a cure. After some research I also knew we were facing a difficult uphill battle, yet after speaking with Dr. Van Dyck and his team, I had hope. Dr. Van Dyck's network was global, he was passionate about understanding this dreadful disease. We were lucky to be accepted into this very sought-after study. It may not have offered a cure, but I hoped it might offer a way for us to hold on to Mom a little longer.

So, in July of 2012, we embarked upon this new adventure together. The study required monthly visits to Yale New Haven Hospital, and Mom and I were starting to get our rhythm established, but it was not without its challenges.

Mom loved rising at the crack of noon. I am a perpetually happy morning person. This was not the best mix. I would be bouncing back and forth like Tigger, rapping at Mom's door promptly at 8:10 in the morning, calling out chipper, good morning greetings. She would grumble about rising early and always had something to say about my jovial demeanor.

About three months into the study, Mom had the luxury of sleeping in until 9:30, that day's appointment was a quick intake meeting with Dr. Van Dyck's team and then we were off to our first MRI. I falsely assumed the MRI would be done at the hospital with that very convenient valet parking, or better yet in the same building as Dr. Van Dyck's office. It was not.

Just when I thought I had all the key addresses for this study mapped out in my head, the team threw me a curveball, telling me the MRI was to be conducted across town. Mom and I climbed back into the car, and I cautiously drove through downtown New Haven, glancing down at the address on the small piece of paper Dr. Van Dyck's intern had handed me. Mom sat in the passenger's seat watching the buildings slip by. I leaned to my right looking out her window for numbers on the concrete buildings when I realized we had arrived at our destination. My foot hit the brakes hard and startled Mom as her seat belt tightened against her chest. I scanned the landscape for a parking lot, only to realize our only option was street parking.

A deep sigh escaped my chest and I hung my head for a moment. This country girl had somehow passed her driver's test twenty-seven years earlier without parallel parking. I had also successfully avoided the terrifying task for two plus decades. That day was the day that streak ended. I blew my bangs out of my eyes with a strong determined puff and squared my shoulders.

It was quite an undertaking, I lined my car up, turned the wheels, and started backing up. All the while with Mom asking repeatedly what I was doing. I tried to tune her out as I attempted to align the passenger side tires with the curb. It took a few tries. My own frustration with my inability to execute a simple driving task coupled with my lack of understanding of Mom's disease made me snap. Her peppering questions got under my skin, and I yelled at her. The minute it happened I wanted to pull the words back from my lips and swallow them whole.

Her response was what prompted my first Facebook post about our journey. It looked simply like this…

Life with MIL…

I parallel parked in New Haven after only eight attempts!

After my second attempt:

MIL: Ummmm what are you doing?
Me: Trying to parallel park.
MIL: Oh…why?
Me: Because there is NO other parking

After my fourth attempt:

MIL: Ummm…what are you doing?
Me: Trying to parallel park
MIL: Oh…why?
Me: (forcing a smile) Because there isn't parking anywhere else.

After the seventh attempt:
MIL: Ummmm…
Me: (screeching) Ma! I'm trying to parallel park and I suck at it!!
MIL: Geeezee, I thought you could do anything.
Me: Sigh

On the eighth attempt we finally parked…I guess I needed her vote of confidence!

The post was a way for me to release my guilt and to share how wonderful Mom was, I never knew it would be the beginning of something very special. The responses to that post were filled with support, love, and comradery that quickly made me realize that this journey of Alzheimer's was touching more people than I ever could have realized. There is a small part of me that sometimes doesn't want to admit that Facebook is where the first story of *Life with MIL* was penned. Think about it, who starts a book on Facebook? Mom and I did.

I

The Awakening

How Do You Spell "Alzheimer's"?

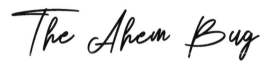

The Ahem Bug

Connecticut

November 2012

The leaves danced and twirled from the tailwind of the car ahead of us. I was mesmerized by the way the sun's scattered rays bounced off the brilliant leaves as they put on a dazzling show, one that could have been choreographed by some of Broadway's finest. I glanced over at Mom. We were settling into our "new adventure" surprisingly well. We were five months in and had already learned so many valuable lessons. I was learning, among other things, how to parallel park and she, well Mom wasn't learning anything, she was just being Mom.

That beautiful performance happening before me on the pavement also brought with it my fall allergies. I always felt lucky that my symptoms were mild, more annoying than anything else. This fall morning, my nose tickled a bit and I found myself repeatedly trying to clear my throat.

Me: (coughing) Ahem…ahem (coughing).
MIL: You okay?

I raised my arm and used the back of my hand to rub my very itchy nose.

Me: Yep…ahem, just got the ahem bug.
MIL: Ahem bug?

Me: Yes, I have fall allergies.

I glanced again over to the passenger's seat and found Mom looking at me curiously.

MIL: Wait, where are you taking me?
Me: To see Dr. Van Dyck and then to Yale for your infusion.
MIL: You should see the doctor for that allergy bug you have!
Me: (coughing *and* giggling) Okay, Mom, but I don't think Dr. Van Dyck can help me.

Smiling, I stole another glance at Mom, her brow was furrowed and she was studying me closely.

MIL: Why?
Me: Well, he's the doctor for the Alzheimer's study we're in.

Mom folded her arms, turned, and settled back into the seat looking out the front window. After a moment she turned back to me.

MIL: I...I think we should ask him; you need him more than I do!

I smiled at Mom and turned to watch the road ahead of me. The bright sun had just slipped behind a dark cloud and raindrops began to spatter the windshield. I took a breath and turned back to Mom.

Me: I certainly hope I don't need him more than you!
MIL: Who?
Me: Dr. Van Dyck.
MIL: Who's that?
Me: (coughing) Ahem...oh, Mom.

Mom turned very serious and motherly as she shook her finger in my direction.

MIL: Don't 'Oh, Mom' me! You should see the doctor.
Me: (smiling) Okay, I will.

Mom, obviously feeling quite accomplished, settled back into her seat with a soft smile on her face. I carefully asked her about the weather, without clearing my throat.

Me: How about this rain today?
MIL: Yep, it's raining.

I smiled and shook my head lightly. Yes, we were settling into the adventure and I was learning along the way.

The Refillable Glass

Connecticut

April 2013

Tuesday night became one of my favorite nights of the week. It was firehouse drill night for Fred, Mom's companion. Which meant we 'Mom sat' (sounds so much better than babysitting!). We had recently come to the glaring realization that she could no longer be alone for any extended period. Joe and I always looked forward to spending this time with Mom. While there were challenges, the blessing of the time spent with her far outweighed anything else.

On one particular night, we were cleaning up after dinner. The dishes rattled a bit as Joe closed the dishwasher. I was scrolling my Facebook feed when I looked across the table at Mom. Her arms are folded tightly across her chest as she watched Joe wipe down the counters. I wondered what was going through her head, her face gave nothing away. I tilted my head with curiosity, thinking, *Are her thoughts truly empty?* This is a foreign idea for me, I can confidently say I have never experienced a blank mind. Even in my most quiet moments something is running through my very busy brain. For a moment, if it was true, I was almost envious. I shook away the thought and returned to scrolling through my Facebook feed. I paused after reading a friend's post and decided to share.

Me: Ma, listen to this. People who wonder whether the glass is half empty or half full miss the point. The glass is refillable.
MIL: That's great.

She looked at me for a moment in silence. Then lifted her chin at an angle away from me, pursed her lips, and breathed deeply through her nose. Leaning forward, Mom tapped the table in front of me.

MIL: Write that down for me.
Me: Okay.

Obeying unconditionally, I stood up from the table, walked across the kitchen, and pulled a sticky note and pen out of the junk drawer. Mom watched me intently as I made my way back to the table. I reopened my phone and copied the words onto the note, carefully and neatly. With the note stuck to the tip of my index finger, I held it up for Mom to see across the table. She pulled the note off my finger, examining the hot pink piece of paper carefully. In classic Mom fashion she curled back her lip a little, picked her glasses up off her nose, and squinted intently.

MIL: What's this?

I tilted my head and thought, *Really? You just asked me to write this down for you!*

Joe smiled as he slid a kitchen chair out from the table and joined us.

Me: Read it.
MIL: (sighing deeply) People...people who wonder...leather the glass is... leather? Ummm, why leather?...leather glass?

I covered my mouth to stifle a laugh. One corner of Joe's mouth started to turn up into a smile as he gently took the sticky note from Mom. He put the paper on the table and patiently pointed at the key words and read. Meanwhile, I wondered how her brain replaced "whether" with "leather."

Joe: Mom, it's whether the glass is half empty or half full.
MIL: (interrupting) Leather?
Me: No, whether, Mom.

Joe leaned back into the kitchen chair, sighed deeply and looked at the ceiling. I started to giggle like a schoolgirl.

MIL: Wait, what's this again? (holding the paper again in her hand)
Joe: Oh my God.
Me: (working hard to contain my composure) Mom, it is a quote from my
    friend Christine, you asked me to write it down.
MIL: Oh, I did?!?

I could no longer hold it back; the laughter crept up the back of my throat, threatening to come roaring through. Maybe it was a result of the stress building up after months of juggling the study and my new company. Or maybe I was kissed by the silly bug. Whatever the reason, I was close to losing it. Joe sent me a stern look.

As the tears started to collect in my eyes, and the uncontrollable laughter was working against me to escape, I watched Joe's stern face and realized, Oh no, he's going to think I'm making fun of her! Just as the thought entered my mind, Joe's face began to contort too, as he fought off his own laughter. Mom looked back and forth between the two of us and our laughter became infectious. Mom shook her head gently, then she snapped it back and her face broke into a wide smile. Her nose crinkled while she wheezed a little as her own voice struggled to deliver a sentence between her own fits of joy.

MIL: I...I...(wheezing) have no idea why we are laughing...but...love...I
    love you!
Joe/Me: (laughter subsiding a bit) Love you too, Mom!
MIL: You're my favorite daughter-in-law.
Me: Oh, I better be! (giggling)

Mom saying I was her "favorite daughter-in-law" had become our thing. Even before her cognitive issues, Mom had other health issues, some serious ones. Those health concerns were often aligned with many doctor visits. Joe had always been her advocate, which in turn made me one also, after all there isn't much we don't take on as a team. Over the years, when it was my turn to attend a doctor's visit, I'd always introduce myself as "Lisa, Rosemary's favorite daughter-in-law" paired with a quick wink and sheepish smile. Mom always responded with a wide smile and a nod. I would come to find in the upcoming years that our thing, my "title" so to speak, would actually become the way she would remember me. My name would often escape her lips, but "her favorite daughter-in-law" seemed to find its way to her tongue, along with a smile that warmed my heart every time.

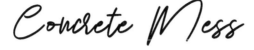

Concrete Mess

Connecticut

July 2013

The state of Connecticut and the city of New Haven had been testing my patience for almost a year. As if life wasn't already serving up its share of challenges, the redesign and construction of Connecticut's Route 34, the exact route we needed to take to Dr. Van Dyck's office and the hospital, seemed to be going at a snail's pace. As I sat in traffic, I'd often remind myself *Lisa, you're not an engineer, don't pass judgment,* but the road work was adding fifteen to twenty minutes to our commute, and, quite honestly, with running my new business, juggling motherhood, household chores, and Mom, every moment was precious! I rolled my shoulders back and leaned into the driver's seat while I watched the brake lights create a red pattern across my Tiffany blue hood. Mom started to fidget a bit, she leaned forward, looking out the front window, then out the passenger window.

MIL: Where we going?
Me: (sighing) To Dr. Van Dyck.

Mom continued to look back and forth through the windows as I scooted up in my seat and craned my neck to see around the van in front of me. I fell back into the seat and looked at the dashboard clock, realizing we were going to be late for our appointment.

MIL: Ppssshhh, yep!
Me: Yep?
MIL: (nodding her head) Yep!
Me: Yep what, Ma?

I quickly glance at her, a little confused. Mom leaned forward again, pointing up to the large buildings, then back at me.

MIL: I'm sure glad I don't live here.
Me: New Haven? Why, Ma?
MIL: I don't know…it's…

Mid-sentence a firetruck approaches the intersection and blows the air horn. I jump a little in my seat. Startled, Mom grabs the dashboard and passenger door. Her eyes filled with fear and her voice was on the verge of shrill.

MIL: NOISY!
Me: (waiting for the fire truck to pass) Yes, it is…but the city has a lot of great stuff too!
MIL: (folding her arms like a defiant teenager) Like what, Smarty Pants?!
Me: (giggling) Did you just call me Smarty Pants?
MIL: (smiling and nodding) Why, yes, I did!

I smiled and shook my head. As the van in front of us started to move, I tried to figure out how to explain to Mom the good the city offered.

Me: Well, it may be noisy, but everything is at your fingertips here. You could live in a city without a car, everything is close…theaters, libraries, stores, restaurants, museums.
MIL: (interrupting me) It's…it's…look at the…(leaning forward again, pointing to the skyscrapers, shaking her finger).
Me: The big buildings?
MIL: Yes…too many people, too noisy…I don't like it here.

Mom sat back in her seat, folded her arms, and set her jaw as I made the turn into the driveway. It probably was too many people for her, too noisy for her. I could only imagine how confusing, even frightening, it must have been for her.

MIL: Humph.

Me: (looking to defuse the situation) Well, Ma, what do you like about where you live?

Mom turned and looked at me, pursed her lips, and rolled her head to look back out the passenger window

MIL: There's not this mess…this UGLY mess!

Me: Mess…hmmmm that's one way to put it.

Mom looked back at me, examining my face. I recognized that she was upset, and I didn't want to bring her into the hospital agitated. My mind started to scramble for ways to redirect her thinking.

Me: Want to know what I like about where we live?

MIL: (snapping back like a defiant teenager) Yeah, what?

I pulled into the valet line, put the car in park, and turned toward her, making certain to have direct eye contact. I smiled and softened my eyes, leaving behind my earlier traffic frustrations.

Me: I like the smell of cow manure in the spring. I love the birds waking me with their songs. I love that I can drive a tractor to pick up Joey at his friend's house and I think it's really cool that when I go to buy a cup of coffee, everyone knows my name.

MIL: It's quiet.

Me: (smiling) Yes, it's quiet and…

MIL: (quickly interrupting me) And Fred's there.

Me: Yep! and Fred's there. We'll get you back to him later today, okay?

The valet approached the car and opened my door.

Valet: Good morning, Madam. Parking for the day?

Me: 'Til at least 2 or 2:30?

Valet: You got it!

MIL: Where are we going?

Me: To see Dr. Van Dyck.

As I walked around to the passenger side, I watched Mom through the windshield, she seemed a little more relaxed, her life with Fred is good for her. A satisfied smile washed back over my face as I reached the passenger side to help Mom out of the car. Then, because God has a sense of humor, an ambulance went squealing by, startling Mom again. I looked to the heavens and shook my head.

MIL: What the hell is that?!
Me: It's just an ambulance, Ma (closing the car door behind her).
MIL: Ppppssshh…Yep!
Me: Yep what Ma?
MIL and Me: (speaking in unison) I'm sure glad I don't live here.

Mom stopped mid-step and looked at me, stunned.

MIL: How did you know I was going to say that?!
Me: I had a hunch.

MIL: Where we going?
Me: (answering as if I'd never heard the question before) To Dr. Van Dyck's study.
MIL: Does Fred know I'm here?
Me: Yes, we'll get you back to him later today, okay?
MIL: (smiling) I know you will. You always do.

I took her hand and guided her up the sidewalk. She continued looking at the tall concrete buildings, very much like a child in the city for the first time. A lump filled my throat. I came to the realization that, as my own children were growing and maturing into adulthood, Mom was spinning backward.

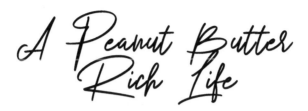

A Peanut Butter Rich Life

Connecticut

August 2014

The grocery bag was slipping down my hip as I opened the back door. I glanced over my shoulder to be certain Mom made it up the back steps of our porch. She was still navigating stairs on her own, despite the grumbling. It was a beautiful late summer afternoon, Fred had asked me to pick up Mom a little early. It was drill night and there was planning to be done for our town's agricultural fair that was coming up. The Durham Fair is a huge event in our town and many local organizations, including the fire house, take the opportunity to raise funds by parking cars.

Me: Come on, Mom, I'll get you settled at the kitchen table while I start dinner.

I leaned back a little in the doorway to see her steadying herself on the top step.

MIL: I'm comin'…(humph)…comin'.
Me: You got it, Beautiful. You're a spring chicken!

I quickly dropped the groceries on the table, my purse on the kitchen chair, and turned back to help Mom through the back door. Corralling the dogs with one leg and a free hand while I guided her to the table.

Me: Here ya go, Ma, you can sit here and visit with me while I start to make dinner.
MIL: Okay!

Keeping the back door open I shooed the dogs outside, the last thing I needed was two dogs sniffing Mom and pushing her buttons. I slid the kitchen chair out and Mom sat with a deep sigh. I delivered a gentle squeeze to her shoulder as I swept the grocery bag off the kitchen table. Mom seemed a little restless tonight. I watched her fidget with a few pieces of mail on the table.

Me: How we doin' over there, Ma? (placing an onion on the cutting board)
MIL: Good?

Watching Mom carefully with one eye, I continued unpacking vegetables. She shrugged her shoulders and turned over an envelope once, then twice, then turned it again and tossed it aside. She repeated this with three more pieces of mail. I wondered if she needed a few minutes of my undivided attention, so I walked back around the counter and over to the table. I gently put my hand on her shoulder and kissed the top of her head.

Me: What can I get you?
MIL: Nothing (sounding dejected).

She took her hand and squeezed mine as it rested on her shoulder, which simultaneously created a very odd crinkling noise coming from her chest.

MIL: Humph?!

Mom looked up at me with great curiosity and, not missing a beat, reached through the neck of her shirt, slid her hand into her bra, and pulled out a Reese's Peanut Butter Cup.

MIL: Wow! Will ya look at that?!

Me: (slightly stunned at what she is producing out of her bra) What ya got there, Ma?

MIL: Well, it looks like a candy!

Mom glanced up at me and smiled. She ripped the package open and was ready to devour the candy, for a moment reminding me of Violet Beauregard from Charlie and the Chocolate Factory. She was almost a little too eager to tear into the wrapper!

Me: (chuckling lightly) Gee, what else you got in that bra?!

Mom stopped opening the package and looked at me with great anticipation.

MIL: I don't know, let's check!

Mom started digging around in her bra, first on the right side then on the left, thankfully she came up empty handed!

MIL: Well, I guess there's nothin'. But! It is a good place to hold important things isn't it?!

Me: (shaking my head and smiling) I guess so, Mom!

Mom sat back in the chair, finished opening the wrapper, and started to bite into the peanut butter cup. Pure joy and bliss washed over her face, her eyes closed as she savored the sweet treat.

I knew she was borderline diabetic. I knew she shouldn't be eating the peanut butter cup. But, life is short. Just moments ago she was fussing, she was clearly agitated, now in the blink of an eye or, better said, the crinkle of a candy wrapper, she was smiling ear to ear. Mom seemed pretty peaceful and content at that moment, so I let that one go.

I gave her shoulder a soft pat, my way of saying I needed to get back to the kitchen. She tilted her head toward me and smiled widely, with chocolate and peanut butter across her teeth, and gave me a quick nod.

As I slid the chicken into the oven, ideas rolled around in my head on what to do with Mom while dinner cooked, and we waited for Joe to come home. Last week she sat at the table while I worked on a few notes for clients. I was totally consumed in my work and not at all paying attention to her, tonight would need to be different. It was a perfect late summer night. There was just a hint of fall in the air. The nights were starting to get a little cooler, yet when the sun started to slip deeper into the sky it warmed the back porch beautifully, making it nothing short of a perfect place to absorb the remnants of the day in peace.

Me: Heya, Ma, I've got an idea. Let's sit on the back porch while dinner cooks, it's a beautiful night don't you think?
MIL: (shrugging) I guess so…

Mom didn't move, I patted her shoulder and encouraged her to follow me. She turned in her seat, grunted, and shuffled her feet into the ideal position to rise out of the chair. With one arm on the table and her other on the back of the chair she took a deep breath and pushed herself off the chair. So often it seems like so much work just for her to stand, I almost want to cheer when she does it without too much effort!

Me: There ya go, Beautiful!
MIL: Yeah…

The screen door bucked and jumped as I slid it open, for a split moment I reminded myself to ask Joe to grease the track. As I stepped onto the porch, I waited to let Mom pass, knowing she'd never be able to handle closing the screen herself.

Me: Have a seat, Ma; we'll sit for a spell.

She rested her large frame into one of our white rocking chairs. As the rocker leaned back, she gasped, her hands grasping the arms of the chair as if bracing herself for the ride. Knowing she'd settle herself, I smiled and watched her. Within moments she was rocking peacefully gazing out upon our backyard.

MIL: (breaking the silent rhythm of the chairs) This your house?
Me: Yep!

Mom nodded and continued to rock. I watched her enjoy the movement and the peace it seemed to offer her.

MIL: (ceasing to rock and leaning forward looking at me) Where's my son?
Me: He's on his way home, he worked today.
MIL: Oh, did you work today?
Me: Sure did, I left a little early to come pick you up.
MIL: Sorry.
Me: No sorrys to be had here, it's good to spend time with you. We have lots of fun together!

Mom returned to her rocking. I put my head back against my own rocking chair and closed my eyes, listening to the rhythmic sounds the chairs made.

MIL: This is a nice house.
Me: Sure is, and ya know what? Joe built it!

Mom stopped rocking, slammed her hands on the arms of the chair, and looked at me with wide eyes.

MIL: (appearing genuinely shocked and surprised) WHAT?! Joe built this?!
Me: (smiling and nodding my head) Yes, he did! Of course, he had help from family and friends, but he built it.
MIL: I knew I had a talented son! (pride beaming through her smile)
Me: (nodding in agreement) Yes you do.

Mom continued to rock. I closed my eyes again and enjoyed the sun on my face. The rumble of my son Joey's truck came up the driveway. I waited for his heavy boots to hit the back stairs. Joey at sixteen was as tall as Joe, he had hands the size of baseball mitts and was a gentle giant. He possessed at this young age the traits of a man well beyond his years. Joey never complained when we asked him to "Grandma sit," this disease didn't scare him. He figured out his own ways to be with her, it isn't what a grandmother and grandson relationship should be, but nevertheless he made it good for him.

Joey: Hey, Grandma (kissing her cheek).
MIL: Hi!?

The sun was falling partially behind the tree line, casting a slight shadow over Joey's face. I was not completely sure Mom was registering who Joey was, she turned to me, looking a little confused. Joey kissed my cheek and headed through the back door, the screen bucking as he closed it. Again I think we need to grease that door track.

MIL: This is your house, right?
Me: Yes, it is Mom.
MIL: (stopping her rocking chair) REALLY?!
Me: Sure is.
MIL: WOW, you sure must be rich!
Me: (chuckling) Rich? Not really, Ma. *Rich* is a relative term.
MIL: (confusion washing over her face) Relative term...huh?
Me: A "relative term" kinda means two people perceive the same word differently.

Mom looks at me blankly, blinking twice.

Me: Trust me on this one, Ma, Joe and I aren't rich...we work long hours to have what we do.

Mom shrugged her shoulders and returned to her rocking. Her soothing tempo is interrupted by the sound of Joe's truck coming up the driveway.

MIL: Yep, you're rich.
Me: I don't know about that.
MIL: (no longer rocking, leaning forward in her chair) You. Are. Rich! (spreading her arms wide). Look at this beautiful house and big yard!

Just as she made the declaration Joe walked up the backstairs.

MIL:...and my handsome son!

Joe leaned down and kissed his Mom. I watch her look at him, she knew who he was and was smiling at him. He stood above her in his uniform and I realized how difficult it must be for him to watch her slipping away. He was in a unique position as a firefighter/paramedic, he had assisted in bringing life into our world and watched others cross over out of this world. He had a different perspective on what was happening to his Mom, he'd watched it for years in various patients and never spoke of the doom and gloom, but embraced and loved what we had right then with her.

Me: Ma?
MIL: (patting Joe on the arm) What?
Me: You are right, we are rich!
MIL: Huh? What you talkin' about?
Me: Nothing, Ma, but thank you.
MIL: Well I don't know what I did, but you're welcome.

Again, she somehow had done it, Mom had a way of keeping things in perspective. I thought of my lessons from Mom that day:

- Your bra is a good place to hide important things.
- Life is short, eat the peanut butter cup.
- We are rich.

The love we share, the life we live despite the challenges and heartache we experienced with this horrible illness, it did have its silver linings. It was becoming crystal clear to me that we would only survive it by remembering how short life is and how rich we are.

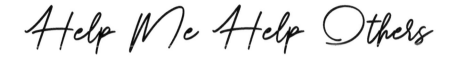

Help Me Help Others

Connecticut

January 2015

I stood at the kitchen sink washing potatoes as Mom sat at the table watching Joey intently.

Me: (watching him work on his homework) Hey Buddy, how's it going over there?
Joey: Okay.
Me: Need a hand?
Joey: Nope.
Me: (shaking off the last potato) Mom, how is he doin'?
MIL: Good!…errrr I think…(chuckling lightly).

I looked over my shoulder at her and remembered the great day we had together. It had been a long day, but nevertheless great. We started very early at Dr. Van Dyck's office for one of her long intake visits as required as part of the study Mom was in. Mom had her vitals taken, her weight recorded, and we updated her long list of medications. Then they swept her into a room for a series of questions and asked her to attempt simple tasks. I sat in the waiting room with my laptop and phone and worked. Then it was my turn to sit through a series of interviews. That day's interviews were done by one of my favorite people, Martha.

Martha: How's she doing, Lisa?

Me: It's been okay. She seems to have plateaued. Is that possible?

Martha: Sure is.

Me: We had a great morning; she was up and ready to go when I got to the house. She even (chuckling) walked out to my car and said, "I love this car, it is the best color!" Tuesday night when I picked her up at the firehouse and was walking out to the parking lot toward my car, I had to redirect her to follow me, she didn't know my car (shrugging). Today she knew the car and was a chatterbox the entire ride from Durham.

Martha: Hmmmm…(smiling and leaning forward just a bit) treasure days like today.

Martha opened a file and took out a stack of papers. I adore Martha, but, I admit, this part of the study was sometimes the hardest. I spent the better part of a half hour answering questions and assessing Mom's progression of this God-awful disease.

Martha: She can complete games and puzzles, well, somewhat well, with help, not at all?

I look down at the table, remembering the crossword puzzle queen now only attempting word searches.

Me: Somewhat well? She won't ask for help.

Martha: Hmmm (glancing back at another page). Is she still doing the word search and Sudoku?

Me: I don't think Sudoku anymore. Just word searches, and honestly those are a struggle.

The questions continued; Martha was perceptive. When she saw my face fall with difficult answers, she would pause and let me collect myself. Her compassion, a warm squeeze of my hand, and her smile kept my spirits up. She even laughed with me when we shared a humorous story.

I returned to the waiting room to find Mom "reading" a magazine. I wish I knew what was happening in that once brilliant mind of hers. In the past, her chair would always have a stack of newspapers and books by its side. She was like a sponge sucking up the words and knowledge.

Me: Hey there! Ready for some lunch before your infusion?

MIL: Sure! Where we off to?

Me: (looking back at Martha and smiling) How about Subway today? We'll get you some fresh spinach on your sandwich!

MIL: Yum (wrinkling her nose and looking at Martha)? Did she really say spinach? Yuck!

Martha: (laughing) It'll be good Rosemary…you'll have fun!

MIL: Yeah, well that's the truth (wiggling her hips left to right and smiling with a mischievous face). This one and me we do have fun! You know she's my favorite daughter-in-law.

Martha: Yes, she is.

Me: We have a lot of fun! We're like two peas in a pod! Mom's Pea 1 and I'm Pea 2! (laughing) Let's go, Pea 1!

We exchanged our goodbyes and wishes for a happy day. Mom and I continued to our lunch at Subway, then to a three-hour infusion back at the hospital and a half-hour follow-up exam. We made our way into the lobby to wait for the valet to bring our car around. I guided Mom to a series of chairs.

Me: Sit here, Mom, I need to give the valet my ticket.

MIL: Okay.

Me: We'll pick up Joey on our way home and then go to our house for dinner. Fred has a firehouse thing tonight.

MIL: Okay (yawning and looking at my computer bag). You didn't work today.

Me: Yeah, I did, while we were at Dr. Van Dyck's and while you had your infusion and slept. Hey! (laughing) Why are you yawning!? You just had a three-hour nap!

MIL: It's hard work!

Me: (shaking my head) Oh, Mom.

The sun was lower in the sky, the days were getting shorter, which meant our moments of clarity were also shortening. As the sun escaped the sky, Mom seemed to slip away with it too.

I busied myself in the kitchen working on dinner, while Mom asked Joey what he was doing.

Joey: (rubbing his face and rolling his eyes) English homework, yuck!
MIL: I used to be a writer. I loved English.

I just about dropped the pot I was holding. Just the other night when I picked her up at the firehouse, I was reminiscing with her and had to tell her she was a writer once.

Me: (filling the pot with potatoes) Mom...
MIL: Hmmmm?
Me: (hauling the pot onto the stove) I've been doing a little writing too.
MIL: Really?
Me: (standing at her side, placing my hand on her shoulder) Yeah, I enjoy sharing our story.
MIL: (turning and looking up at me) Us? You mean you and me?
Me: Yep! I love telling people about our adventures (biting my bottom lip a bit), and honestly how you and I are navigating this new life you've been handed.
MIL: New life? (tilting her head)
Me: Remember? (gently tapping her forehead) This beautiful brain of yours seems to be short circuiting. That's why we go once a month to Yale?
MIL: Oh, yeah...it's called...(holding her forehead and squeezing her eyes shut tight). What's it called?
Me: Alzheimer's...it's called Alzheimer's, Mom.
MIL: Yes that's it.
Me: So. Mom?
MIL: Yeah?
Me: About my writing...
MIL: Oh yeah! Let me hear about it ...
Me: Well, it involves you and I...

MIL: Really? (sitting back in her chair and smiling) Tell me.

I opened my laptop, opened my Facebook page, and started scrolling through my *Life with MIL* posts and reading them to her. The early ones were pretty funny, and she laughed along as I read them, then I read a more serious one, and I stopped and looked at her. There Mom sat, staring at the kitchen table. I searched her face for some kind of answer on how she felt, but her face was unreadable.

Me: Mom?
MIL: Hmmmm?
Me: You okay?
MIL: Uh huh…
Me: You sure?
MIL: Yes…I am. (She looked up and leaned in close to my face) These are good…really good.
Me: But sometimes it's not funny or pretty…
MIL: This thing I got (tapping her forehead) this…is…
Me: Alzheimer's?
MIL: Yes…others have it too, right?
Me: Yeah, Mom, too many people have it. That's why so many people can relate to our stories. Lots of people reach out to me and tell me our stories are comforting, they don't feel alone and sometimes they find a different way to handle the disease.
MIL: Hmmm…
Me: Hmmm what, Ma?
MIL: (leaning close to me with determination and intensity in her eyes) Don't stop, keep going…it may be the only way I can help others.
Me: That's pretty brave, Mom. We don't know what the future holds.
MIL: No, I don't…but I know this…I know you can help me help other people.

I reached across the table, pulled her close, and just held her for a moment. I sat back in my chair and looked across the kitchen table at Joey. He had abandoned the English assignment and was just watching us. I wondered what he thought of the last few years. He as well as my daughter Ashley had lost the grandmother they had grown to love so much. I was proud of both of them in how they handled this new reality of life with Grandma. I tussled Joey's hair as I made my way back to the kitchen.

Joey: Grandma?
MIL: Yeah?
Joey: Tell me a story.
MIL: Hmmmm. Whadya want to hear?
Joey: I don't know, you choose.

I don't remember what story Mom told that night, it was probably something about her father's blacksmith shop. Memories of her childhood seemed to be popular at the time. I do remember standing in the kitchen listening to Mom talk and heeding Martha's words, "Treasure days like this." That day was a treasure, for more than a fleeting moment I had Mom again. I often reflect on that day; it was the day she urged me to continue telling our story. Remembering her insistence, the intensity and passion in her eyes, face, and voice helped me continue through this very difficult journey, and so I treasure that day.

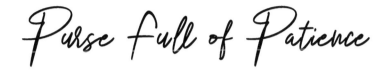

Purse full of Patience

Florida

February 2016

It had been a grueling few days. I had two intense deadlines at my Connecticut studio, the stress of this was exacerbated by Joe's desire to leave by 1:00 p.m. on Thursday to embark on the drive to Florida. We drove straight through twenty-four hours from Durham to Naples only to arrive on Friday afternoon to no bed to sleep on at our destination.

Two months previous, Joe had successfully found us a one-bedroom apartment in central Naples. There would be no more suitcases and hotel rooms for me, or us! LDD's second location was no longer "a thing we were trying," it was a reality.

Then came the task of furnishing an apartment, I had forgotten how much stuff you need to set up home. We spent two days shopping, hauling furniture, boxes, and multiple bags up and down a flight of stairs; it took a toll on both Joe and me. We were exhausted both physically and emotionally yet fueled by the excitement of this newest chapter. At times I found myself feeling like a giddy newlywed again.

Then the phone rang.

Joe: Fred! How are ya?

I stopped opening the new sheets for the bed and walked four short steps into the living room. Fred had recently purchased a home in Florida, outside of Daytona Beach. He and Mom had begun the trips south the previous winter in search of this second home. I had often expressed my concern about Mom being so far away, but Joe had reminded me that the sun and longer days would be good for her. I tried to remind myself that I, too, was frequently traveling between Naples and Durham, and while this new home was five hours northeast of our apartment, it was closer than it was to Durham. I was beginning to think we'd be making that trip sooner than expected.

Joe: Yep.

I intently watched, absentmindedly folding the sheet packaging as my heart rate climbed just a bit. Joe was staring at the floor, chewing the inside of his cheek. I listened to his side of the conversation.

Joe: So when are you heading back?…Okay, we're in Florida ourselves.…No, driving.…Tuesday…Sure.

Joe smiled a little and looked up at me. Our gazes connected.

Joe: Hi Ma!…It's Joe…Ma? You okay?

The smile quickly faded as a cloud crossed his face.

Joe: You're breathing awfully heavy, is anything…huh?

I walked closer, Joe shook his head.

Joe: Ma? Can I talk to Fred?…Fred, she okay? She's out of breath and huffin' and puffin'…chased by a dog? What?

There was concern in Joe's eyes and he was doing that thing with his jaw that makes the muscle flex in his cheek. I truly began to worry.

Joe: I don't know…let us see how much we can get done here. You sure she's okay?…Yes, Route 4, I think it's about four and half hours…yep…Fred, Ma's okay?…Yeah.

Joe hung up the phone, squatting as he put it on the floor. He rested his head in his hands.

Me: Honey? She okay?

Joe: I don't know, it sounds like she can barely catch her breath, she was pretty ornery. Fred says she's fine. They're heading back to Connecticut in two weeks.

Joe let out a long sigh and scrubbed his hand over the top of his head.

Me: We can leave really early Tuesday and spend a few hours there, see if we can get a good assessment on how she's doing…

Joe looked up at me, I knew the look; he needed to see her right then. I looked around at our little apartment, the dinette area was filled with boxes and stuffing four feet high. I sighed, thinking this would all be waiting for me when I returned by myself at the end of the month. How could I do all that by myself if we left that day? I squatted down next to him and put my hand on his shoulder.

Joe slapped his hands on his lap and stood up.

Joe: We gotta get you more settled.

Me: Honey…if we gotta go, we gotta go. I'll figure it out.

Joe: Maybe you call Fred in a little bit, maybe he'll tell you how she really is.

The worry in his eyes, worried me.

Joe: Let's just keep at this.

I waited about a half hour, probably the longest half hour we'd experienced in a very long time, before I called Fred.

Me: Hi Fred! It's Lisa!…Yeah…beautiful eighty-four degrees here today, uh huh…tired but good…

I walked into the bedroom, Joe didn't follow.

Me: Fred? Mom didn't sound so good when Joe talked to her a little while ago, how she doing?

I listened as he told me she was fine, that she had just walked in from getting the paper with him. A dog had barked and startled her, so she was more winded than usual. I asked how she was doing otherwise. He continued that she had her moments, but they were doing just fine. He suggested I talk to her to see for myself.

Me: Hi, Ma!
MIL: Well, hello!
Me: You know who this is?
MIL: Ummmmm…yes?
Me: It's your favorite…
MIL: Oh! My favorite daughter-in-law! (giggling)
Me: How you feeling Ma?
MIL: Oh, very good how about you?

On the other end of the phone I heard a very relaxed, chipper, and breathing-normally woman.

Me: I'm good…Joe and I are in Florida too!
MIL: You are?. . . Fred? Am I in Florida?
Me: Yes, you are, Ma…would you like us to stop and say hello on our way home?
MIL: Oh, I'd like that!
Me: Me too, Ma, it's been too long since I've wrapped my arms around you.
MIL: Good.

We said our goodbyes and hung up. I held the phone, looking for a place to put it among the boxes, then turned to find Joe. He stood leaning against the kitchen counter. As I entered the small space, he shrugged his shoulders and looked at his feet.

Joe: She sounds good huh?
Me: Yeah, she does. Maybe it really was nothing. Fred said it was just a dog that scared her.
Joe: Humph.

I studied his body, it spoke volumes. He was carrying a load of concern that would only be lifted by seeing her with his own eyes.

Me: Fine or not, we'll leave early tomorrow to go visit. Not that she'll remember (giggling lightly), but I did promise to wrap my arms around her.
Joe: (smiling softly and letting a chuckle out himself) Yep, and she'll be so surprised to see us!

Joe and I left at sunrise the following day to drive to Daytona to check on Mom. It was a beautiful drive across the state, God has a neat way of making some things just a little more tolerable just when you think they can't be. We arrived early in the afternoon, and Fred greeted us in the driveway. Mom didn't really move from her chair.

Joe: Hi, Ma!
MIL: Hello?
Me: Hey ya, Beautiful!
MIL: Hi?

We know she has no idea who we are.

Joe: It's me, Ma, Joe, your son.
MIL: (a little clarity flittering across her face) Hi…(a smile creeping in)
Me: Hey…you know me…
MIL: Oh?
Me: I'm your favorite…
MIL: (her eyes brightening) Wait! Don't tell me…

33

Mom looks to the ceiling.

Me: Yep, I'm your favorite…
MIL: Daughter-in-law!

I leaned in and kissed her forehead. Her hair was a knotted mess, her teeth desperately needed to be cleaned. Guilt flooded my body. I knew Florida was good for Fred, I knew in some ways it was good for Ma also, but there was just stuff she couldn't do for herself anymore.

Joe and Fred chatted about the house, and we started the penny tour. I tried hard to not focus on the dirt and dust but rather watch Fred's proud face as he showed us around.

Mom sat in the front room staring at the television. I touched her shoulder and she jolted away from me startled. I smiled and stroked her arm gently… she stared back blankly.

Fred: Rosemary! Whadya say we take the kids for a ride and show them some sites?
MIL: Well, okay…(appearing a bit dejected)
Joe: Come on, Ma, it'll be fun…we can see the Garage…

Mom struggled to get out of the chair. She stood and shuffled, huffing and puffing as she made her way to the kitchen. She stopped midway and turned to me, clearly confused.

MIL: Where am I going?
Me: We're going to take a ride.
MIL: Oh.
Fred: Here's your sunglasses, purse, and hat.
MIL: I don't want those.
Fred: Take them anyway…you'll want them.
MIL: (sighing) No I won't (more defiant now).

Fred waved his hand and walked away. Mom definitely tested his patience at times. I often wondered how their relationship worked. Mom knew Fred from high school, he had been Joe's father's best friend. The best friend she admitted she didn't care for at all, even calling him a bully and troublemaker. Decades later, at a high school reunion, ironically less than a year before her diagnosis, they reconnected. I would discover through the years that their relationship was one of companionship and convenience. Fred certainly cared for Mom, and I believe she gave him purpose. Although I doubt he ever knew the weight her illness would carry.

I looked at Mom holding the hat, purse, and glasses. Like a child she put the hat on. She opened the purse and put the glasses inside. The only thing in the purse was a stack of tissues. She closed the purse and sat at the kitchen table.

MIL: What's this for? (holding up the purse)
Me: We're going for a ride, your purse has your glasses and tissues…you're going to want those.
MIL: Oh, why?

I studied her carefully. My mind wandered to a memory of her sitting at my kitchen table years ago.

She had just come back to Connecticut for a visit from Arkansas. Ashley was about seven years old and she was reading to Mom. Her face was filled with concentration and her blonde hair was stacked upon her head. She was struggling a bit. Mom patiently guided Ashley without judgment, she didn't show frustration when Ashley repeatedly missed the same word. Instead, she found a way to redirect her and taught her to "see" the words another way. Mom celebrated Ashley's successes with laughter and kisses. Ashley struggled for another few years but then became an avid reader. That kid would devour books like ice cream on a hot August afternoon, less the brain freeze. No, her brain didn't freeze, it grew in leaps and bounds and she became a well-rounded woman. This was no doubt due to the seed that Mom planted.

I was snapped back from my memory when Mom asked yet again what we were doing.

Me: We're gonna go for a ride, Fred and Joe are getting the car ready.
MIL: Oh, what's this? (holding up her purse)

I remembered the judgment-free zone at my kitchen table with Ashley as I squatted down in front of Rosemary. I gently placed my hand on her purse and took it carefully anticipating a great surprise.

Me: Well, let's see whatcha got in there?

I looked up into her blank eyes and winked. I opened her purse quickly, then snapped it closed.

Me: Phew, that was close!
MIL: (now intrigued and leaning forward) What?
Me: I don't know if you want to know what's hiding in there! (shaking my head with faux fear and anxiety)
MIL: (giggling) What, show me! (smiling)

I thought I saw her eyes dance for a minute. I slowly opened the purse revealing the pile of tissues and sunglasses.

Me: (squinting my eyes closed) Go ahead, you're brave…you look!

Wails of laughter rolled from her lips. I opened one eye.

Me: Is it safe?
MIL: You're so funny, I love you.
Me: I love you, too. Let's go for that ride. When we get back, I'll brush out your hair. Would you like that?
MIL: Yeah! Where are we going?
Me: To see the sights…it'll be fun.
MIL: Okay.

I took her hand and guided her out through the garage. Fred and Joe waited in the driveway, the old Chrysler had its top down, and a light breeze swayed the palm trees gently behind them. Fred tapped the hood gently and said something about taking the "ole girl out." Mom laughed and adjusted her hat. As we backed out of the driveway, I saw Mom's reflection in the side view mirror. Her chin was lifted toward the sun, the corners of her mouth turned up slightly, she was clearly content. The miles between us were hard, they were scary. I often wondered if the trips were worth the stress and anxiety it caused, yet maybe they were good for her.

The Hairdo Strut

Connecticut

April 2016

I was struggling to maintain my positive demeanor. Joe had sent a text earlier that day letting me know he was taking an overtime shift that night. I was admittedly frustrated, it was Tuesday night, which meant we were Mom sitting. I had been hoping to sneak back to the studio to work for a few hours but instead I brought the work home and decided to do what I could at the house.

I made the short trip from the studio to Mom's house and picked her up. We enjoyed a nice dinner and now as I was cleaning up, my mind was creating a list of all the things I needed to complete tomorrow morning. I snapped the lid of the last Tupperware container closed tight. Balancing the stack of leftovers, I turned toward the fridge. I glanced over at Mom who was watching my every move from the kitchen table.

MIL: Your hair…how do you…(touching her head with her fingertips) ya know, how do you get it to…(pointing back at me)…humph.

Me: (closing the fridge) How do I do what, Ma?

MIL: Do THAT! (pointing at my head) Your hair…to do that?!

Me: I don't know, Ma, I just do it? (running my fingertips over the top of my hair)

MIL: I need to do that…I need to go to…to see a…a girl.

Me: We can do that.

I made a mental note to try to get Mom into a salon this weekend, there was no time during the week. As I closed the dishwasher, I looked over the counter at Mom, she looked so distant. The dishwasher kicked into its wash cycle as I made my way to the table.

Me: Come on, Ma, let's get you cozy in the family room…I'll ask Joey to change what he's watching.
MIL: No, no…let Joey watch his stuff…

She struggled to stand but gained her balance. As she turned to the family room, she stopped abruptly.

MIL: I'll use the bathroom first.
Me: Okay.

I left Mom to take the short trip to the bathroom on her own. The distance from the kitchen table to the bathroom door is no more than half a dozen steps, how much trouble could she get into? I settled into the sofa and picked up my computer.

Me: Joey, let Grandma watch the game shows.
Joey: Yuuuup.
Me: Thank you.

Mom entered the family room, and we started our routine "to get cozy." This was when I would set her up on the sofa, feet up on a stool, pillows behind her lower back as well as her head, and a cozy blanket over her. This entire process took five minutes, or more. It was a repetitive list of demands: "The pillow isn't right. Pull the stool closer…not too close. Humph…can you move the pillow?". This task alone was enough to exhaust even the most seasoned caretaker never mind this gal whose mind was on the consultation notes I needed to complete. I kissed Mom's forehead and returned to the sofa. I picked up my computer and quickly became engrossed in my work as Pat Sajak welcomed that night's guests.

MIL: Humph…
Me: Yeah, Ma (not looking up from my computer).
MIL: (throwing the blanket aside) Humph…how does she do that?!
Me: (still looking at the computer) What, Ma?
MIL: THAT! Look at her!
Me: (still engrossed in my work) Okay, Ma…

I was so involved in my notes I didn't even realize Mom was restless. She let out a loud grunt, shuffled herself to her feet, and started to leave the family room.

Joey: Where ya goin', Grandma?
MIL: Bathroom…

Hearing Joey's comment, I looked up to discover Mom wasn't sitting on the sofa across from me. I had been so concentrated on my work, I hadn't heard her get up. Trying to keep an ear on what she was doing but still make some headway on my notes, I turned back to my computer.

A commercial break came across the television and Joey headed into the kitchen. He returned with a second glass of milk and another stack of Oreos. I thought, *That kid has a hollow leg!* Then I suddenly realized Mom had been gone awhile.

Me: Grandma is still in the bathroom?!
Joey: Yuuuppp.

I put the computer down and started to get up from the sofa when Mom entered the family room. She had a strut to her walk that was well, almost sexy. Her petite frame carrying over two hundred pounds was swinging her hips from left to right. One hand was on her hip while the second stroked back her hair. She wore a smile of confidence and accomplishment. I watched in confusion mixed with a healthy dose of amusement.

Me: Ma? What did you do to your hair?
MIL: What? (stroking her fingers through her hair again) You had some of
    that fancy hair stuff…the sticky stuff…I thought I'd…(twirling her hand
    over her head) I fixed the mess!

41

I look at her blankly for a minute. I was scrambling to figure out what she could have put in her hair, after all she was only in the powder room.

Me: Hair stuff?
MIL: Yep! (closing her eyes craning her neck to the right, she sets her jaw with smirk of triumph)

I realized at that moment that Mom must have taken the liquid hand soap and used it as hair gel. I looked down at Joey, who just stuffed an entire Oreo in his mouth, and mustered every ounce of composure I could find.

Me: Ma? That was not fancy hair stuff, that was hand soap.

Joey looked up at me, his eyes popped open as he studied me for a nano second. He couldn't contain himself, he spit Oreo and milk all over my coffee table as he broke into a fit of laughter. I worked hard to contain my own amusement, and seeing Joey's reaction, as messy as it was, definitely wasn't helping.

I walked toward Mom and placed my hand on her arm. Realizing she thought she looked amazing, I needed to tread lightly.

Me: Come here, let me clean you up (still trying to keep a straight face).
MIL: (clearly confused) What?
Me: You just have to add a little water to it, it always is a tricky formula.

I took Mom into the bathroom and rinsed her hair the best I could. I then combed her wet hair, which, with the weight of the residual soap, was no longer falling in her eyes.

Me: There...better?
MIL: (looking at me and squinting her eyes) How you do that?
Me: Do what, Ma?
MIL: THAT?! (pointing to my head)

I shook my head and kissed her forehead.

Me: Mom?

MIL: What?

Me: Thanks for always making me laugh.

I turned her toward the mirror.

MIL: (her eyes widening as she smiled) Well, look at THAT! You did…(pointing to her head) you did THAT!

As I helped Joey do a final clean-up of the Oreos and milk, Mom tried to get herself resettled. I offered my help and again it took many tries before the pillows were just right and the stool was not too close but not too far. By the time I opened my computer again she was snoring away. Looking, I might add, pretty stylish.

This journey was filled with fun times. We didn't take every situation as a catastrophe, keeping in mind that soap and Oreos can be cleaned up, and these times would make for great memories someday.

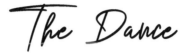

The Dance

Connecticut

August 2016

The past few months brought to the surface a few new challenges for us. During a recent interview with Dr. Van Dyck's team I shared that Mom no longer seemed to be able to clean herself and we'd noticed occasional incidences of incontinence. Martha asked about household tasks, and I hung my head and shared that those, too, were becoming more and more difficult. I didn't like admitting Mom was slipping away, although Martha always had great insight on how to keep her active and engaged. So that was exactly what we did, we added housekeeping and weekly showers to our adventure.

I snapped the top bed sheet and watched it float effortlessly down over the mattress, it nestled itself perfectly across the bottom bed sheet. Mom stood across the bed in total amazement.

MIL: Wow, you're good at that!
Me: Pppssshhh, I've been making beds for years, Ma.

I quietly and mindlessly tidied and smoothed the top sheet across the bed. As I finished, Mom pulled the opposite corner toward her. My perfectly centered and masterly laid top sheet was now filled with wrinkles.

Patience I tell myself.

I picked up my side of the top sheet and tugged it toward me, straightening the wrinkles as I did so. With a quick tilt of my head, I examined the side of the mattress, satisfied with the equal distribution of the sheet, I turned to grab a pillow as I heard Mom fidgeting.

MIL: (holding up the side of the top sheet) How much you got?
Me: I'm good over here Ma, about the same as you.

I started to make my way to her side of the bed to straighten the top sheet, again.

MIL: How you do that?
Me: What?
MIL: That...do that so fast!
Me: Make the bed?
MIL: Yeah.
Me: (leaning my head to the right and shrugging my shoulders) I don't know I just do.

I lifted the comforter over the top of the bed, shook it out, and watched it fall into place. As I straightened a few buckles in the fabric, we engaged in another mild tug of war. I came out the victor, as Mom finally just surrendered the comforter and watched as I finished.

Me: There! How's that, Ma? Fresh sheets, and now onto this mess!

I dropped a very full laundry basket onto the bed.

MIL: Why you doing that? (her face full of question)
Me: Doing what...folding the clothes?
MIL: If that's what you call it!
Me: (giggling and shaking my head) Because we can't put crumpled up clothes in the dressers. Everything will be a wrinkled mess!
MIL: Oh...okay...

It almost appeared to be a foreign idea to Mom, this household task, one that while she was raising five children on her own had to be a daily chore. In my own mind I questioned how folding laundry could be something she didn't know. She had to know it, like she knew to take a breath to breathe!

I watched her as I held up a pair of underwear and easily and quickly folded it into a neat square.

MIL: Do that again
Me: Fold the underwear?
MIL: Yeah…show me how…

I picked up two pairs and handed one to Mom. Carefully I walked her through, step-by-step, how to fold them. She folded down when I said fold left, she crumpled when I said smooth, and when I placed my neat little underwear square in the pile, she laid out a ball of underwear.

MIL: Humph…(defeat falling like a dark cloud over her face)
Me: Not bad, Ma! Here help me with this one.

I took her ball of underwear and smoothed it out on the bed. Then standing next to her, I took her hands and slowly guided her through the steps, creating a neat (perfect, actually) little underwear square.

MIL: Better…(a proud smile skating across her lips)
Me: Yeah, better than mine!
MIL: (giggling) Yeah it is!

The tasks continued, t-shirts folded, pants neatly stacked. I quickly paired a few socks, tossed them aside and sighed as I dumped out a pile of mismatched socks.

Me: (spreading the pile of socks across the bed) Ma, see if you can find the ones that go together.
MIL: (looking skeptical but determined) Okay…ummm…okay…

She slowly picked up a sock and examined it thoroughly. I turned and started to inspect her dresser drawers and found myself pleasantly surprised. Each week I typically found a mess, a wreck of dirty clothes mixed with clean clothes topped off with discarded Kleenexes and maxi pads in her drawers. Tonight, the drawers held mostly clean clothes.

Me: Your drawers look good, Ma!
MIL: Oh?
Me: Uh huh! Really good, nice job!

I looked over my shoulder as I was delivering her compliment and found she was holding two red socks, one narrowly striped, the other solid. She was intently studying the two, I could almost see the wheels turning in her head as I watched her.

Me: How you doin' with those socks?
MIL: I know these go…(studying the socks closely), but they don't…(looking at me, inquisitive) do they?
Me: (smiling warmly) Nope, they don't, but they sure are close though, don't you think?

Holding out the two socks Mom passed them off to me, I dropped the solid red sock and quickly picked up the coordinating striped sock. In a swift effortless motion, I tuck one sock neck inside the other and cast it aside into the pile of paired socks.

MIL: (sighing) How you do that? (looking dejected)
Me: Pair the socks?
MIL: If that's what you call it…(frowning)
Me: Well, first I lay them out nice and flat so I can see them clearly, then match them up! Let's be fair, Ma, in this pile you only have a couple of matches left. Here, let's find them together, okay?

Playfully we sorted through the pile, occasionally I adorned Mom's head with a colorful sock pretending it was a glorious hat! Laughter was a wonderful remedy for a dejected spirit. We found three pairs among what had to be over two dozen odd socks. Three pairs, that was another small victory tonight! I placed the unmatched socks back into the laundry basket, with the hopes that next week some of their matches would magically appear.

Mom stood watching me. She held her right hand over her left, absentmindedly stroking her right thumb over the left. I made a mental note to paint her nails the following week, that would be a fun release.

Me: You just about ready for your shower?
MIL: (confused) Why, where we going?

Our first shower night was when Mom and Fred had a dinner to attend, so she then assumed whenever I assisted her that she had some place to go.

Me: Nowhere. It's just bath night!
MIL: (shrugging her shoulders) Well, I guess so…
Me: Good, hang tight, I'll let Joe know we're getting in.

I walked down the hall to tell Joe we were getting in the shower shortly. He smiled at me from his mom's recliner. His face was full of gratitude, love, and a hint of guilt, he was often apologetic when chores like showers fell on my shoulders. He need not be, while Mom often tested my self-control, it was an honor to care for the woman who gave me such an amazing man.

This journey continually threw me curveballs I was often unprepared to catch. This night, my return to the bedroom offered a new surprise as I pushed the pile of dirty sheets out of the way to close the door. I heard it before I saw it. It was the mumbling that caused me to turn, there I found Mom digging aimlessly through a pile of clothes on the bed, one dresser drawer open and another just about empty. She mumbled incomprehensible phrases as she pushed her hands through the pile of clothes. I reminded myself to dig deep and find some patience. Washing over me was a mix of feelings ranging from frustration to anger to defeat, but mostly sadness. Mom had no idea we had spent the last hour tiding up her room and dresser. I crossed the room, clearing my throat so she knew I was back. I placed one hand on her left shoulder and my chin on her right. I tilted my head toward hers and asked with caution…

Me: Ummm, what ya doing there, Ma?

MIL: I don't know. These need…(quickly and forcefully dropping her hands at her sides)

Me: Need to be put back in your drawers? Did you empty your drawer?

MIL: (shrugging) They just need…

I sigh. This was our dance. I'd put the clothes away and she'd dump them out. I'd make the bed, she'd pull and wrinkle the sheet. I looked to the heavens and asked for restraint and poise.

Me: (starting to refold the clothes) Okay, Beautiful, we've got to get in the shower.

MIL: Oh? Where are we going?

Me: Nowhere, it's just bath night (placing the last shirt into the drawer).

Me: You start to get undressed and I'll warm up the shower.

MIL: Okay (looking through the pile of mis-matched socks).

I stepped into the bathroom and started the shower. I put out the towels and return to the bedroom. There was Mom, leaning against the bed…blowing her nose in a sock. I watched her for a minute, she rolled the sock in her hand, opened the top dresser drawer, and dropped it in. My shoulders dropped; my heart hurt for a moment. She didn't see or feel the disappointment or temporary frustration washing over me, and I thank God for that small favor. I closed my eyes for a moment, breathed deep through my nose, and allowed the air to escape through my lips slowly. I smile and step toward Mom, guiding her to the bathroom.

Me: All set, Ma!

MIL: What…What are we doing?

Me: Showering. Come on in, I've got the shower warmed up!

MIL: Where we going?

Me: Nowhere, it's just bath night. You know, the night where I scrub your back and wash your hair.

MIL: (eyes lighting up) Oh, I like that!

Me: (chuckling) You certainly do.

While Mom stepped into the bathroom, I opened the top dresser drawer, pulled out the sock that recently took on the personality of a Kleenex, and tossed it in the pile of dirty clothes. Then I stepped through the bathroom door and looked at Mom standing in the bathroom staring back at me.

MIL: Where am I going?
Me: (sighing) Nowhere, Ma, it's just bath night (as I kiss her forehead).

I turned and closed the bathroom door, and our routine began. First, I hold out the bowl.

Me: Drop 'em in, Ma!
MIL: What?
Me: Your teeth.
MIL: Oh (dropping the dentures into the bowl).
Me: Thanks! (acting as if she just gave me a dozen red roses) Go ahead let's get undressed!

I watched her as she undressed. She looked up at me and, for a moment, love radiated from her eyes.

MIL: Whaf fould I do wif out you?
Me: (giggling) I don't know, Ma.
MIL: Fank you.
Me: (giggling) Can you keep talking to me? I love how you talk without your teeth, it's so funny.
MIL: Hey! You're a braf!

I kissed her forehead again. Our time together was precious. I am not a home health aide, and, honestly, some nights I didn't want to be taking care of these tasks. It could be frustrating and exhausting. Somehow though, every night I was with her, at some point, she seemed to have a moment of clarity and would tell me how much she appreciated me, loved me, or would ask, "What would I do without you?" The back and forth, the round and around each night with Mom was our dance. When I thought of it this way, it was actually somewhat enjoyable. I hoped I would continue to see those times as just that...the dance.

51

MIL: (looking in the mirror as I comb out her hair) Where am I going?
Me: Paris!
MIL: Whaf?
Me: (laughing) You're not going anywhere Ma. It's just bath night.

Round and around we go…

I Need to Ask a Question

Connecticut

October 2016

Drill night arrived like it did every Tuesday, but this week it seemed to sneak right up and bite me on the backside. When Fred called earlier with my reminder to pick Mom up, I was caught off guard, I had forgotten it was Tuesday. Joe was working a day shift so I thought I had at least a few extra hours to work at the studio. Deadlines were looming, I was leaving for the Florida office soon, and every moment was precious. Nevertheless, I responded to Fred's call with my typical cheerful response and quickly buttoned up my day to drive the few short miles to pick Mom up.

I didn't realize until we were all gathered around the dinner table that I needed a break from work. It was nice to have Mom and Joey at the table. Although I was missing Ashley (she was living in New York City at the time), it was shaping up to be a nice evening. The sun had set behind the tree line, dinner dishes were cleared, and Joey had slipped into the garage to tinker on his truck. Joe had arrived home a few minutes earlier and he, Mom, and I sat around at the dinner table making small talk.

MIL: I need to ask you a question (a look for confusion clouding her face).
Me: Sure, Ma.

She seemed hesitant, tracing a square on the table with her fingers.

MIL: There's a…(squeezing her eyes shut in concentration)…you do this…
Me: Ma? What do you mean?
MIL: (sighing) I don't know how to explain it…(tapping her head)…it's stuck.
Me: (a wave of compassion washing over me) I know, Ma…
MIL: Never mind

I looked at Joe who was staring at the table. It was amazing how fast the atmosphere could change. I scrambled to bring back the relaxed feeling we had just been experiencing.

Me: Do you know what Joe and I did Sunday?
MIL: No…
Me: We had so much fun. We dug through an old barn for a client, let me get the pictures…
MIL: Okay.

I grabbed my laptop and started scrolling through pictures, showing Mom the old milk buckets, hay rakes, and more. Joe began to share stories of his youth, when he and his brother Scot worked on a local farm, just up the street from where we sat.

MIL: (leaning in to look at the computer) Where's this?
Me: Middletown.
MIL: Oh…Humph…I…I have…(squeezing her eyes shut again) I need to ask you something.
Joe: Go ahead, Mom.
MIL: It's a piece (drawing a square on the table with her fingers)…kinda of paper you write on…
Joe: A note?
MIL: No, well…kinda…but kids do it.
Me: Kids?
MIL: Yeah, you write on it and…give it to someone.

I looked at Joe confused. Then I realized this must be the "sundowning" I had read and heard about. The team at Yale had shared that sundowning is a common experience for people living with Alzheimer's disease. The patients experience increased confusion, anxiety, and even disorientation that starts around dusk.

MIL: I don't know, but I should have done it because I just left work…They don't know where I am…they aren't going to pay me.…

Joe looked at his mom, then at me, then back at his mom. She was clearly entering a moment of warped reality. Did she think she was at Pratt & Whitney, the aerospace manufacturer where she used to work as a technical writer? I wondered if she punched a time clock during her time there. Either way, she was confused and clearly very worried. Joe slid his arm across the table, gently taking her hand in his.

Joe: Mom, it's okay, you're retired.
MIL: No, I'm not…and I didn't…(tapping her head) leave it…the thing…
Joe: Mom (looking at her with so much compassion my heart begins to break).
MIL: What?
Joe: It's all okay.
MIL: But I didn't leave (tracing a square on the table again)…
Me: Mom?
MIL: What? (looking at me blankly)
Me: (thinking maybe we just enter her reality with her) Where are you working?
MIL: Down the street.
Joe: Mom (taking her hand), you're all set you're retired.

Mom sat back in the chair with a little force, her face was blank as she folded her arms tight against her chest. Joe and I locked eyes for a moment. I didn't like the feeling in the room, it was unsettling, it was disconcerting, and I needed to change it. I returned to the pictures, flipping the computer screen back to Mom.

Me: This is one of my favorites…
MIL: Where's this?
Me: Middletown.
MIL: Oh.

Joe followed my lead and continued with more memories of Joe and Scot on the farm. I smiled, laughed, and enjoyed hearing the stories, some for the first time! I wondered if Mom knew them also, or, if she did, did she remember them? She laughed and seemed engaged, but as quickly as she was captivated by Joe's stories, we lost her again.

MIL: Can I ask you a question?
Me: Of course, Ma.
MIL: There's a thing…(squeezing her eyes tight). You write on it.

Joe rose up from the table and pulled out a stack of Post-it Notes and index cards from the junk drawer. Mom was tracing squares on the table again.

Me: A note?
MIL: No…yes? You write on it…kids…(tapping her forehead).
Joe: Like this Mom? (showing her the index card)
MIL: No! (emphatically)

Joe then took the Post-it Note and began to write on it.

Joe: Is it a Post-It Note you're looking for? 'Cause you can write a note and stick it someplace to remember or remind yourself of something.

Joe then stuck the Post It Note to his forehead, it said, "I LOVE MOM." I giggled and shook my head lovingly toward Joe. I watched Mom as she sat back in her chair then leaned forward again, looking intently at Joe's forehead, clearing trying to read the note.

MIL: No…it's a…like a paper you, pass it…like kids

Joe studied his mom for a moment, then took an index card and began to write on it. He folded it neatly and held it up.

Joe: Like passing notes in class?
MIL: I…I ?
Joe: Here, look, I wrote a note. If we were in school, I'd pass you this and ask you to answer.

Joe passed the folded index card to Mom, inside it said, "I like Lisa. Do you think she likes me?"

MIL: (carefully reading the note) I like Lisa.
Joe: (eyes dancing with mischief) Do you think she likes me?
MIL: Yeah…
Joe: Then you write, "Yes."

Joe handed Mom a pen. She smoothed the index card out and stared at it for a moment. She was concentrating hard but couldn't form the word "yes." She formed a c and two e's.

MIL: (sounding frustrated) I can't…
Joe: It's okay, Ma.
MIL: I need to ask you a question…

Joe and I exchanged a glance. I felt a lump rise in my throat. This was a woman who was salutatorian of her high school class, she easily completed the *New York Times* Sunday crossword puzzle in a morning, yet today she couldn't even compose the word "yes."

Me: Sure, Ma.
MIL: (tracing a square) It's a piece…a thing you…
Joe: Mom, we've been talking about this for the last few hours on and off. Lisa and I can't grasp what you're asking.
MIL: (looking down at the note and picking up the pencil) I think I used to be smart.
Joe: Oh, Mom, you did some great things! You wrote technical manuals for aircrafts; you were an editor for a newspaper in Eureka Springs…
Me: You ran a great little shop called "Weird Sisters" and you dabbled in photography, even did a photo shoot for an emerging country artist's album cover!
MIL: (leaning forward, eyes wide and a smile crossing her face) I did all that?
Joe: Yep!
MIL: Wow! I was smart…
Me: You still are very smart, Mom (gathering her hand in mine).
MIL: You think so, huh?

Me: (looking to Joe and back at Mom) Yes you are. You are teaching us lessons and helping us put life in perspective more than you can ever realize...we call it *Life with MIL!*

MIL: Hhhmmmm (smiling)...well, glad I can do that for you.

Mom sat back in her chair, looking content. I looked at Joe, his face was red, his eyes looked tired to me. I took my free hand and squeezed his hand. I didn't know the unique pain his heart must have been feeling, I did know that he would not be alone on this journey, we would get through it together.

MIL: (sighing deeply) Can I ask you a question? (tracing a square on the table)

Joe's eyes got wide, he started shaking his head, looking down at the table-top and laughing. He lifted his head and looked lovingly across the table at his mom.

Joe: Sure, Ma, ask away.

Thanks, Mom, for this night, it was a difficult little tango we did, around and around we went about the "the square." It was so much more than that, though. Together I learned and you relearned (even for a moment) stories of Joe's childhood, of the history that shaped the man we so dearly love. As difficult as this journey was, it also presented beautiful moments too. I loved Joe's note, and I'm so glad Joe likes me!

Phone Call Coverup

Florida

November 2016

The sun peeked over the rooftops as I walked to the car. Its rays peaked through the palm trees, creating jagged slivers of light. I was extremely thankful for daylight saving time. I had just scored an extra hour of sleep! I slid across the seat of my rental, opened the convertible top, and set the GPS. I had four and a half hours to go if I didn't stop. I sighed, weighing the reality of what my day was going to entail.

The warm Florida sunshine and wind swept across my face, I sipped my coffee and reflected on the previous day's call to Fred and Mom to finalize arrangements for today.

Fred: Hello?!
Me: Hi, Fred! It's Lisa, how are you?!
Fred: Oh, the phone told me it was you. We're just visiting friends at the Garage.
Me: Aww, that's nice. Fred, I'm thinking I should make it to you around noon tomorrow, how does that sound? I'll shower Mom and visit for a bit.
Fred: Yeah, that sounds good, we'll be here.
Me: Great, I'll call when I'm about thirty minutes away.

*Fred: Here, here's Rosemary (shuffling). Say hello, Rosemary…
no, hold it like…yeah, there ya go.*
MIL: Hello?!
Me: Hi Ma! How are you?
MIL: Great! How are you?
*Me: Good, good! I'm coming to see you tomorrow. Would you
like that?*
MIL: Yeah !

*I could almost feel her smile through the phone. I paused, and
thought, She sounds great. I could hear other people in the background. She didn't seem flustered, anxious, or confused as she so
often was when she was in public places.*
Me: Great, Mom, enjoy your day! I love you!
MIL: I love you, too (shuffling again). Here take this…

I heard Fred talking to someone else as he disconnected the phone.

As my GPS announced an upcoming turn, I started thinking that maybe Joe was right, maybe the sun, warm air was good for Mom. It certainly seemed like it when I spoke with her on the phone. She was happy, upbeat, and, well, good. Could it be that my concerns with her being in Florida were just me being overprotective?

The ride was long and lonely but I was encouraged by the previous day's call. Five hours and fifteen minutes later, I pulled into the driveway and parked the car. I opened the car door, stood, and stretched. Fred was in the front window, watching for me. A light breeze rustled the leaves of the palm tree, welcoming me as I walked to the door.

Fred: (opening the door) Hey there. Be careful, Toodles has been trying to escape all morning.
Me: Hi, Fred. Now, Toodles (pointing a scolding finger at the large black cat), no escaping.

I walked through the door, stepped over the cat, and saw Mom sleeping in the chair in front of the TV. Fred and I made eye contact and he shrugged. I walked around the front of the chair, Mom's hair was a mess and her shirt was on inside out. A soft sigh escaped my lips as I squatted down and gently rubbed her leg.

Me: Hi, Mom!

Mom jumped a little, and her eyes flew open. I could tell she was confused and startled.

MIL: Hello?
Me: Hi (rising for a kiss). How are you?
MIL: I don't know (squinting her eyes and glaring hard at me).
Me: Well, you look good, Beautiful! (rocking back on my heels)!
MIL: Grumph...(waving a dismissive hand at me).

I knew this too well, a kiss on her forehead, a stroke on her cheek, this usually calmed her. It almost seemed to center her. As I did so, I turned to Fred.

Me: How we doing today?
Fred: (sighing) Well...

I looked down at Mom, her head was turned toward the window and she had returned to dozing. I noticed her hair was a matted mess on the back of her head. I squatted down in front of her chair and softly placed my hand on her arm.

Me: Mom?
MIL: What (not opening her eyes)?!
Me: I'm thinking we should get out for a bit today.
MIL: Grumph.
Me: I'll give you a shower, wash your hair and teeth real good...you'll feel so fresh and rejuvenated!

I rubbed her arm to attempt to rouse her. She opened her eyes and glared at me.

Me: Okay! (smiling) I'll go get things ready for us. I'll be back for your teeth in a minute.

I looked up and Fred had left the room. As I headed down the hall, I found him in his office, leaning against the doorjamb. I inquire about Mom.

Me: Hey, how is she today?
Fred: She's tough today.
Me: Did she sleep okay?
Fred: She wasn't up as much as she usually is…she's just, you know…tough.

There was a hornets' nest brewing in the next room, I could feel it. Yesterday's conversation from when they were at the Garage, a local bar, played back in my head. Mom had seemed good. Then it clicked, she had probably been having a few Twisted Teas. Mixing alcohol with this disease can be a nasty cocktail, I was sure we were experiencing the fall out today. I started to ask how much she drank the day before, but decided quickly it wasn't worth the effort. I was certain Fred would see it as overstepping and judgmental. In his mind he believed he knew what was best for her. I pushed my shoulder off the door frame and shook my head in my own private disappointment.

Me: Let me get her showered and cleaned up, then how about I treat you both to lunch. I'm starving!
Fred: (never looking up from the desk) Yeah, I guess…
Me: She seemed good yesterday when I spoke with her on the phone.
Fred: Yeah, maybe.
Me: Well, let me get this going. I should plan on being back on the road by 3:00…sound okay??

Fred nodded. He showed me to the bathroom where we gathered shower supplies and her toothbrush, keeping the conversation light. He showed me to the bedroom, where we found clean clothes. I pulled out a few crumpled tissues and a fresh pair of Depends. I took a deep breath and returned to the living room.

Me: Okay, Beautiful! Let's get this show on the road (doing a little twist of the hips as if we're going dancing).
MIL: What?!

Mom jumped and grabbed both arms of the chair, her eyes wide and a bit wild.

Me: Shhh, shhh, shhh. It's okay, Ma, I didn't mean to startle you! I've got the bathroom ready for your shower, okay?
MIL: Why?!...WHY?!
Me: Because we need to clean you up a bit.
MIL: (staring hard at me) Humph! I guess...

Clearly irritated, Mom pushed hard off the arms of the chair to rise.

MIL: Why am I doing this? (huffing) Are we going somewhere?
Me: Well, I thought after your shower we could go for a late lunch, my treat.

She shuffled her feet as she moved toward me. She was clearly struggling to steady herself. I held out my hand for assistance if she needed it and she waved it away. We struggled through the shower, the space was about a quarter of the bathroom back in Connecticut. It was tight for just Mom to be in there, never mind throwing me into the mix too. This shower day was different than others. For the most part, by the time I got to washing her hair, even on her worst days, her attitude had softened, but not this time. I finished dressing her and hung up the towels.

Me: How about you sit in your chair while I brush out your hair?
MIL: (glaring at me over the top of her glasses) Why?

I leaned in and kissed her forehead, reminding myself that gentle acts of affection always softened her difficult temperaments.

Me: You'll be more comfortable in your chair.
MIL: (snarling) Why are you doing this?
Me: Doing what, Ma?
MIL: (setting her jaw and sending me a shot with her laser eyes) THIS!... this...the...

Me: I love you, Ma, and I know you need the help.

MIL: Humph…

Me: It's us, Mom, you and me getting through this mess called life together.

Mom gave me a partial smile. She grunted and grimaced as she struggled to stand. I walked behind her as she shuffled down the hallway to the living room and collapsed in her chair. I decided I'd let her sit for a bit while I finished cleaning her teeth and the bathroom. I stuck my head through the doorway of Fred's office, and I told him I was just about done. He nodded, shuffling through his papers.

I returned to find Mom sound asleep in the living room. I tenderly stroked her arm to wake her.

Me: Hey there, Beautiful. Time for me to brush out your hair.

MIL: Huh?

Me: There you are! I'm going to brush out your hair.

MIL: (sighing) Okay…

Fred entered the living room and watched me with his hands on his hips.

Me: Did you decide on lunch, Fred?

I concentrated on the "rats' nest" (as my mom used to call it) in Mom's hair. These snarls were becoming a regular occurrence with her more sedentary state.

Fred: You don't holler for her like you do me!

MIL: Whaaaat?! (eyes wide and surprised).

Fred: You yell like crazy when I do your hair…

Me: Aww, Fred, I've got years of experience with Ashley's ha…

MIL: What are you talking about?! (whipping her head so fast toward Fred that I almost brush off her glasses).

Me: Easy, Ma…

I placed my hand on her shoulder and looked over at Fred. He shrugged and pulled the corner of his mouth into a frown. I finished up Mom's hair and patted her shoulder. Fred suggested we sit outside for a bit before we headed for lunch. Mom was reluctant but agreed. I pulled one chair into the sunshine while Fred and Mom sat in the shade, side by side.

For years before Mom and Fred reconnected, he had been traveling down to Daytona Beach and had made many friends and connections. When he and Mom purchased their home here, she did her best to fit in. That day, Fred and I made small talk about how the area had survived the hurricane and how their friends had fared. Mom just stared off into the distance, she barely had anything to contribute anymore to our conversations. Fred suggested we head out to lunch so we slowly made our way to the car. Every other step caused Mom to grunt and scrunch up her face as she expressed her discomfort.

We arrived at Fred's choice for lunch, a local Chinese buffet. He rattled off his favorite dishes as the hostess seated us. I guided Mom to her chair as Fred's phone rang.

Fred: Uh oh. Who's calling? Oh (smiling widely) it's your son!
MIL: Who?
Fred: Hello?...Yes! Hey!...Uh huh...well, we're just sitting down with your mother for lunch here at the buffet....No, Wednesday...(chuckling)...no, we decided to stay through the weekend....Lisa's here...yeah, oh ya know, I told Lisa to tell you, I just saw flights to Daytona from there in Bradley for $249 if you want to come...uh huh...yeah...here, say hello to your mother.

Fred tapped Mom on the shoulder, handing her the phone.

Fred: Here, talk to David.
MIL: Huh? (taking the phone and briefly looking at it)
Fred: Just hold it and talk into it.

Mom stared at the phone, not seeming sure what to do with it, then raised it to her ear.

MIL: Hello?...Yeah, I guess so!...I am?...Yes. Hmmm. Yeah.

A switch flipped. Mom's voice turned pleasant, upbeat, and even endearing. Her face was softer and I saw a glimmer of old Mom.

MIL: Okay…uh huh…love you too…bye bye.

Mom pulled the phone away from her ear and looked at Fred. He quickly took the phone and returned to his conversation with Dave. As he talked, a dark cloud drifted across Mom's face, quickly obscuring that glimpse of sunshine I saw. I realized she still had the ability to fake it. Early in the progression of this disease, family members thought Joe and I were overreacting to her declining cognitive health. I saw now how a phone call like mine the day before or the one I just witnessed would put a question into anyone's mind. The exposure Joe and I had was different, very much like the outburst Fred experienced. We got our own fair share of them. I suspected, because Fred wanted to keep Mom with him as long as he could, he didn't share the dark side of the disease with many people.

As Fred finished the call with Dave our waitress approached and asked to take our drink requests. Fred quickly ordered an unsweetened iced tea, I did the same, then the waitress looked at Mom, waiting patiently.

MIL: (waving the waitress away) I don't know what I want!
Me: Would you like iced tea too, Ma?
MIL: (squinting hard and snapping) I…SAID…I don't know what I WANT!

I jerked my head back from her outburst, but quickly recovered and looked at the waitress and smiled.

Me: We'll think about what she wants.
MIL: I don't know…

The young waitress quickly moved away from the table and I stroked Mom's hand. I looked at her staring at the table and wondered what happened to the woman who just talked to Dave on the phone. I made Mom a plate, cut her food up, and slid the plate and fork toward her. She looked at the fork for a moment, picked it up, and started to use it to eat her lunch. As I watched her, I realized she was only using the fork for half the food she was eating, the other half she was picking up with her fingers. I realized it was taking all of Mom's concentration to just eat her lunch, so I didn't attempt to engage her in conversation. She paused on occasion and looked at Fred or me with confusion or a deep scowl.

As we finished up our plates, our waitress placed the check and three fortune cookies on our table.

Me: Oh fun! Fortune cookies!
MIL: Huh? What's that…
Me: A cookie with a message…or your fortune
MIL: Whaaaat?

Ma said this while raising her voice with a mouth full of food, causing some of it to fall onto her shirt. I leaned across the table with a napkin and cleaned up her shirt.

MIL: Oh, thank you.
Me: it's nothing.

Fred opened his cookie and ironically had a fortune about travel, their plans were to drive back to Connecticut in three days. Mom's fortune gave Fred and I a chuckle, it was about patience.

Fred: What did you get?
Me: (attempting to create a little anticipation and fun) Oh it probably says I'm perfect in every way and people will want to be me (giggling).

Mom glared across the table. I smiled and blew her a kiss. She rolled her eyes at me and sighed. Then folded her arms across her chest and glared at me. I cracked open the fortune cookie and slid out the message. I swallowed hard…

Fred: Whadya got?
Me: Your example will inspire others.
Fred: Nice.

I looked across at Mom as the death stare continued. I knew I didn't deserve the outbursts or the dirty looks, it would be so much easier to just not deal with her. Yet I also know she didn't even know she was doing it. If she did, she'd be mortified. I realized again how much I miss her.

Me: Mom? (giving her hand a gentle squeeze) You just about ready?
MIL: I guess…

On the ride home Fred took the scenic route, sharing their "other hometown" with me. Mom stared out the window, offering nothing to the conversation. When we arrived back at their house, I helped Mom out of the car and got her settled in her chair. I watched as she almost instantly drifted off to sleep again. Fred and I chatted for a moment more about their upcoming trip home. When I looked at the clock, I realized I had to get back on the road myself.

Me: Mom? (gently rubbing her hand)
MIL: Huh? (eyes half open and groggy)
Me: I'm leaving.
MIL: What?
Me: I love you and I'll see you when you get home.

Mom closed her eyes and drifted back off to sleep.

I sat behind the wheel of the car and looked back at the house, Fred was standing in the door waving goodbye. I raised my hand, waved, and put the car in reverse. I reached the stop sign at the end of the road and turned right. I accelerated the car and let the sun and breeze dry the tears that started to slide down my cheeks. The wind felt good on my face as I relived the visit in my head. I had been so encouraged by my conversation on the phone the day before with Mom. She had seemed so…good. I understood, then, that those phone conversations were just an act. It was amazing, and disheartening, to watch her flip an internal switch to be someone else on the phone.

I was about a half hour into my trip when I decided I was going to need coffee. I still had five hours ahead of me and the weight of the day was heavy on my mind and body. I pulled into a coffee shop and walked in to place an order. When the coffee was ready, I opened my wallet to pay, smiled at the young man at the register, and scooped up my coffee. I started to walk away when I was called back.

Cashier: Excuse me, Ma'am?
Me: (stopping to look over my shoulder) Yeah?
Cashier: You dropped this. You might need it.

He smiled and held a small piece of paper that had fallen out of my wallet. He began to read it.

Cashier: Your example will inspire others (smiling and handing it to me).
Me: Thanks…I do need that.
Cashier: Drive safe.

As I slid behind the wheel, I smiled and thanked God for acknowledging my good deed today. He had sent an angel to redeliver the fortune cookie message to me. He knew the struggle. It sure felt good to feel His love, it also gave me far more of a boost than the coffee could ever do.

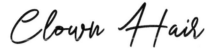

Clown Hair

Connecticut

December 2016

The weekly routine had been weighing heavily on my shoulders, my company was growing and doing well, which meant my travel schedule was starting to become more regular. Joe and I had floated the idea of a home health aide to help, but it had fallen on deaf ears. Fred seemed to feel we could handle the current state of affairs and, more importantly, he didn't want a stranger in his home.

On this particular Saturday, I had blocked off my morning to help Fred and Mom with more than just a bath. I arrived at their house and headed to the door. Fred opened it before I could even knock. I flashed a warm smile, hoping to soften the tough exterior armor he so often wore.

Me: Hey, Fred!
Fred: She's upstairs.
Me: (instinctively knowing something is not right) How is she?
Fred: Well...ya know (hanging his head and walking toward the stairs).

I followed Fred and noticed the stairs needed to be swept. Piles of cat hair and dust had accumulated in the corners. I sighed and a wave of guilt flashed over me. I thought how I should make an effort to do more cleaning than just the bedroom.

At the top of the stairs the sun streamed through the large windows, shadowing Mom's face. There was an uneasiness in the air, I took a deep breath and forced my eyes to dance and smile.

Me: Hi, Mom!
MIL: Hi?

I got a little closer and saw the blank look on her face.

Fred: We were just having breakfast, want coffee? Here sit for a bit (pointing to a chair next to him).
Me: Okay…Mom, how you doing today?
MIL: Okay.

Mom looked at me, studying me for a hot moment, and then looked quickly away. I knew she was trying to register who I was. Fred and I made small talk while I occasionally glanced back at Mom, watching, waiting. *It'll come.* I hoped. If I was patient, she would connect the dots and realize who I was.

Fred: Yeah, so we've lost some shoes and I don't know what's going on with her clothes.
Me: It's fine, should I start with the closet?
Fred: Yeah, we didn't get to that last time…start there, that's good.
Me: Good, and how about a shower? (looking at Mom, crinkling my nose) I think we need to do a shower.

I looked at Mom. I tilted my head and squinted my eye…nope nothing yet.

Me: Mom? How about a shower today? I'll wash your back, give your scalp a good scrubbin'?!

There it is! She made the connection and smiled at me.

MIL: Yeah! That be nice!
Me: It will be…we'll go through your clothes today too…maybe find some shoes?
MIL: (shrugging and pointing at Fred) I don't know…where's my shoes?

Fred: I don't know...where's your shoes? (flailing his arm out, pointing across the room) You take them off everywhere!

Mom shrugged and started stacking the breakfast dishes. Fred and I headed to the bedroom to assess today's project. Piles of clothes are on her dressers and side chair, five mismatched shoes are neatly lined up in front of the closet, the bed is neatly made but the room needs to be vacuumed and dusted.

Fred: Well, I'm trying (pointing to the shoes). Here's what I've found so far... and this (pointing to the piles), I'm not sure what she's done, clean, dirty...
Me: (putting my hand on his arm) I know Fred. I'll clean it all up

I sighed, we returned to the kitchen to find Mom holding the cat food dish, standing in the middle of the kitchen. She's staring at the dish.

Me: Mom? Whadya doin'?
MIL: Ummmmm...
Fred: I'll do that, Toodles's food is here (reaching for the upper cabinet).

Fred sounded frustrated and in need of a break. He took the bowl, and Mom walked toward me, shuffling her feet and hanging her head. She understood she'd been dismissed.

Me: Mom? (sliding my arm over her shoulder) Want to be my helper?
MIL: Sure! (smiling) What are we doin'?
Me: Cleaning your closet and dressers! (giving a little fist pump into the air) Wahoo! Sound like fun?
MIL: (smiling and giggling a little) When has cleaning ever been fun?

There she was...she was coming back to me.

Me: It's always fun with me!

As we walked to the bedroom, I wondered if she would understand what a mess she had created.

MIL: Oh my...I guess I did make a mess.

Me: Nothing we can't fix (kissing her forehead).

Mom sat on the bed. I gave her a pile of mismatched socks to keep her busy as I started in the closet. I sorted clothes, shoes, miscellaneous empty shopping bags filled with tissue, and more. Then I found a clown wig. I knew humor and laughter was as good for her as it was for me! I pulled the wig onto my head over my baseball cap and turned to check on Mom.

Me: How's the sock matching going?
MIL: (not looking up from the pile) Not well…well, maybe these go…(holding a light blue and light green sock together)
Me: Not quite…they're close but they don't match.
MIL: No? (looking up and knitting her eyebrows)
Me: Nope.
MIL: Ummmm…
Me: (purposely acting like nothing is different about me) Yeah, Ma?
MIL: Ummmmm what did you do to your (pointing to her head)? You don't (her face is confused)…that's not your (pointing to her head again).
Me: (giggling) What, don't you like it? It's very colorful. I think it might be a good look for me…maybe I'll wear it tonight to the firehouse dinner.
MIL: (bursting out laughing) I like it!

We sat on the bed laughing. I asked her if we should see if Fred would notice. She gently pushed me and laughed harder. I loved that she could understand the joke that day.

I continued to work in the closet, pulling out sheets and blankets that belonged in the linen closet and finding all but two shoes. Fred poked his head in to let me know there was a load of laundry in the dryer.

Me: I'll have more soon…but I'll wash them, no worries.

I turned to look at Mom. I made a funny face and pointed to my head. She started to giggle.

Me: Fred, notice anything different about me?
Fred: Oh, yeah, that's a good look (chuckling)

MIL: (laughing) Yeah it is!

Fred shook his head and turned to walk away. I stopped him and told him I'd clean the bathroom before I gave Mom a shower. He thanked me, looking at the floor. I fully realized he didn't want to admit he needed the help, which just fed into my frustration toward his resistance to hire a home health aide. When I had tried to talk to Joe about it, he said, "Mom seems to be happy. Fred and Mom have a special companionship. Right now it's not perfect, we'll just keep doing our part. It's best for Mom."

I opened Mom's top dresser drawer where I found more mismatched socks mixed with wrinkled shirts, underwear, various folded and crumpled paper towels, and a few sanitary napkins.

Me: Oh my, I think we need another garbage bag, how about you, Mom?
MIL: (leaning over and looking into the drawer then up at me) Maybe?
Me: (bending down and putting my nose to hers) I think so…unless you have
    a use for crumpled, used tissues and paper towels?
MIL: (crinkling her nose, smiling, and shrugging) Maybe?
Me: (giggling) Maybe NO!?

We rubbed our noses and laughed. I turned to leave the room, telling mom I'd be right back. I returned to find Mom on the bed intensely working at the back side of a sanitary napkin. As I approached the bed, she peeled the back off the napkin, exposing the adhesive.

Me: Ma?
MIL: (jumping, startled) What!?
Me: Sorry I didn't mean to scare you but…what are you doing?
MIL: I need to take this off so I can blow my nose, you know my nose is al-
    ways…(tapping her nose). I need to blow it…
Me: Oh, Mom, not with that.
MIL: (looking quite annoyed) Why not?! I need to blow my nose!
Me: (placing my hand on hers and handing her a tissue from the dresser) Mom,
    here's a tissue…this (taking the pad from her) will stick to your face if you
    try to blow your nose into it!
MIL: (staring blankly) Oh…

Me: (leaning into her face and smiling) Unless, of course, you want a pad stuck to your nose! We'd make quite a pair—you with a maxi pad on your face and me with this hair!

She threw her head back and laughed. This particular crisis was averted, and I was relieved her moods had lately been changing faster than the direction of the wind on a blustery October day.

We finished her dressers, pulling out almost two more loads of dirty laundry. It had already been a lot, with closet organization, cleaning dresser drawers, folding laundry, and laughing at clown hair. She was showing signs of getting tired, and a little cranky, so I suggested a nap while I cleaned the bathroom. She was asleep in her recliner moments after she leaned her head back.

I gently rubbed her shoulder a couple hours later.

Me: Hey, Ma! Ready for that shower?
MIL: (groggily) I guess…where, what…where am I going?
Me: The firehouse dinner tonight!
MIL: Okay…Did you tell me that already?
Me: (thinking, *Only a dozen times.*) Nope, I think I forgot.
MIL: (smiling and shaking her finger at me) I think you did…I think you probably told me a lot, but you won't admit it…
Me: (putting my finger to my chest, looking innocent) Me? Do something like that? I wouldn't do that!
MIL: Yes, you would, and you do (holding her head high).
Me: (kissing her forehead) Well, I do on occasion, but not today.
MIL: Really? It's okay if you did.
Me: I know.

I left after four and half hours, I kissed her cheek and told her I loved her. She smiled, ran her hands through her hair, and told me she felt great.

Me: See you tonight.
MIL: Really? Where?
Me: Firehouse dinner.
MIL: Oh, did you tell me that already?

Me: Nope I forgot.
MIL: Oh good!
Me: (winking) Love you!
MIL: You know you're my favorite…
Me: I know.

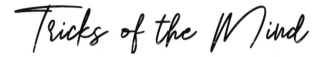 Tricks of the Mind

---

Connecticut

May 2017

Tuesday night dinners had become a steady routine. When this added responsibility of drill night first fell upon us, I wasn't really sure we could do it. Yet, we were doing it, and we were teaching valuable lessons to our children along the way. Ashley and Joey were witnessing and, more importantly, becoming active members of Mom's care.

I have often said, "If you want to hear God laugh, tell him your plans." This new life we were living had never been in my plan, but the journey that was laid out before us was building precious memories. All of us—Joe, the kids, and myself—were learning lessons and building a history that unbeknownst to us would only make us wiser and give us a unique perspective on life. The kids had already proved this on many occasions. They showed the compassion, empathy, and patience that was often not found in their generation, and they prioritized family.

Lost in my thoughts, I pulled the saucepan out of the lower cabinet and knocked over the rack of lids, sending two of them crashing onto the floor.

MIL: (almost jumping out of her skin) What the hell was that?!
Me: Sorry, Ma, I dropped the lid.
MIL: (confusion clouding her voice) Oh…ummmm? I…I…

Me: Yeah? (replacing the lids on the rack) Ma, you need something?
MIL: I…Oh…

Distress was filling her voice, I turned around to see her squinting her eyes and tapping her forehead.

Me: You okay, Ma?
MIL: I want to tell you something…

Her focus was so intense. I left my cutting board and walked to the kitchen table, she was clearly distraught.

Me: What is it, Ma? (gently placing my hand on the top of her head and stroking back her hair)
MIL: I…I…(tapping her forehead again) Oh, I don't know…I can't seem to get it out.

I studied her for a moment as the back door opened and Joe walked through the mudroom. I squeezed her shoulder, my way of giving her gentle reassurance and I allowed my eyes to connect with Joe's. We had honed the art of an unspoken conversation; he read my face and stepped in without missing a beat.

Joe: (leaning in to kiss his mom) Hey, Ma!
MIL: Oh! (smiling up at him and seeming to forget for a moment what was distressing her) Well hello there!
Joe: How ya doin'? (stroking her back lightly)
MIL: Good!

Joe, without even changing out of his uniform, pulled out the chair next to Mom. They made small talk as I finished making dinner. The conversation drifted from Joe's drive home to the dogs wanting to go out the back door and back into the mudroom a few times. Then, suddenly that unsettling cloud returned to Mom's face.

MIL: (looking at Joe very intently) I…ummm…geezzze…I…
Joe: What, Ma?
MIL: I…I want to…(her face twisting into a grimace) No…I…I don't know.

I started to set the table for dinner. I was pleased Joey would be joining us for dinner that night. He was a chatterbox lately, life was exciting for this young man. As I suspected, Joey delivered through dinner, he shared a story about a friend's truck and something about tires and mud. He and Joe laughed while they talked shop. I shook my head often, not truly understanding everything they were discussing! I made eye contact with Mom, widened my eyes and raised my eyebrows. Then I rolled my eyes as a smirk turned up the corner of my mouth. Mom smiled back and shrugged, then started digging through her dinner.

Joey finished, scraped his plate clean, and announced he had to leave for the fairgrounds. He was dedicated, putting in countless volunteer hours preparing our local fairgrounds, which hosted our hometown's pride and joy, the Durham Fair, Connecticut's largest agricultural fair. One of Joey's favorite places at the fair was the farm museum filled with antique machinery and memorabilia. He got up, put his dishes in the sink, and went over to Mom, where he leaned down and kissed her on the top of her head.

Joey: Bye, Grandma!
MIL: Oh…(looking up to Joey confused) bye?!
Joe: He's going to the farm museum.
MIL: Oh…(jumping slightly at the slamming door as Joey leaves) I…umm…I
    don't know…I…(pursing her lips).
Me: (sliding my hand across the table to hold hers) What is it, Ma?

I was growing concerned. She was obviously upset about something she couldn't put into words.

MIL: I want to tell you something and I'm not sure…I don't know…
Joe: Take your time (stroking her arm). What is it?

Mom sat back in the chair, folded her arms, and looked to the ceiling. Her jaw was clenched tight as she closed her eyes. Joe and I exchanged a look, both wondering *What is this?* Thoughts raced through my mind. *Why does she look so scared? Has someone hurt her? Is she okay?*

MIL: (leaning forward wringing her hands) I need to tell you…

Joe: Go ahead, Mom.

MIL: (sighing) You know I was homeless (Mom's eyes filling with tears)…I was living in an old empty house with no food, electricity…it was dark, and I was all alone…

I sat stunned, watching Mom for a moment. I turned to reconnect with Joe, but he was looking at the table. His jaw was set, there was a vein in his forehead that began to pulse as he started to shake his head slowly. I watched as the muscle in his jawline flexed, as his face became more and more pink. I was at an absolute loss for words. I knew for a fact that what Mom said wasn't true. She was delusional.

Me: (looking from Joe to Mom) Where were you, Ma?

MIL: Well…I don't know…it was cold and dark. I was…scared and very lonely (sighing)…but then Fred came and saved me.

I looked at Joe as he took his mother's hand, his eyes filling with tears. While Fred offered Mom a lot, Joe had always taken responsibility for his mother. The youngest of five children, Joe always stepped up to be her caretaker. She relied on him to decipher and be her second set of eyes and ears in all aspects of her well-being, a duty he proudly took on. It had to cut deeply to hear her say she believed she had been left alone.

Joe: Ma, you were never homeless.

MIL: Yes, I was…I remember it (her eyes intense, her hand slapping the table hard)…it was…it was…cold…cold and dark…

Joe: Mom. I love you. I would never allow you to be homeless! Me and Lisa would have you here with us if you didn't have a place to live.

MIL: No? But…I can…I know…

Mom shook her head and looked down at the table. When she looked back up, tears were filling her eyes. She quickly returned her stare to the table.

MIL: I remember Fred getting me!

Joe: Mom, (voice cracking) I can't have you believing that…I'm sorry…I just can't.

The pain on Joe's face was almost too much for me to handle. I struggle to understand why Mom would think this way.

Me: Ma? Look at me...

Mom looked up from the table

Me: Sometimes...sometimes things get a little mixed up in your brain...
MIL: I know...I...

Now tears are welling in my eyes. Not only can I see the pain in her eyes, but I feel it, my heart physically hurts.

Me: Ya, know how sometimes you can't find the words for things? How sometimes you can't remember what you had for lunch?
MIL: Yeah?
Me: It's because you have an illness...Alzheimer's...
MIL: Oh. Yes...
Me: Well, with this illness sometimes things get messed up in your memory. You weren't homeless and alone.
MIL: But...
Me: (cutting her off before she can continue) You may have felt alone in your heart a while ago and then Fred came into your life and then you felt fuller, but you were never ever cold and hungry. Your mind is creating a warped sense of reality.
Joe: Ma? Really, I would never allow that to happen ...
MIL: Oh...it's just...I was...
Joe: I love you, Ma.
MIL: (looking at Joe) I love you too. I know you love me.

Mom reached across the table for Joe's hand and held it tight. He leaned down and kissed her hand. Watching the two of them was heartbreaking. We had experienced times when Mom was confused, when she asked about who was watching her kids for example, but never anything quite like this. There before me sat the woman who years ago raised five kids on her own, wrote aircraft engine manuals, was a lousy cook but an amazing writer, and now was entering a world of warped reality.

Me: Come on Ma, let's get you cozy.
MIL: Huh?
Me: Let's set you up on the sofa.
MIL: Okay...Where's Fred?
Joe: He'll be here soon.
MIL: Oh...good.

Joe helped her out of the chair. I grabbed the pillows, blanket, and stool and started the process of fluffing pillows and adjusting the stool, knowing it would take a few tries to get it just right.

MIL: (sighing) This is nice...thank you.
Me: Love you, Ma.
MIL: Love you too.

Mom placed her head back against the pillow, closed her eyes, and smiled. I hoped there were no more thoughts of being homeless. Joe watched her from the other sofa. There was a sadness I couldn't fix, and the reality that this was only the beginning.

Cost? Hug and a Kiss

Connecticut

August 2017

The television blared from across the room at Fred's house as Mom gently rocked in her chair. The nightly news was reporting the latest updates on North Korea as I stood in the kitchen slicing beets.

MIL: Humhdmlghsnng (incoherent) What are they *talking* about?
Me: Just the news, Ma (continuing to cut beets).

Mom sighed heavily, shaking her head. Dusk, which often delivered a volatile personality from Mom, was upon us. I rinsed the next beet and picked up the knife. As I sliced through it, the blade hit the cutting board with a solid strike.

MIL: Are you washing my dishes?
Me: Nope! I'm making you beets, Ma!
MIL: Beets? What the hell are *beets?*
Me: Those red round things I brought you and Fred from my garden Sunday.

Mom stared hard at me. I could almost feel her anger digging deep into my soul. She let out a deep sigh and abruptly turned in her seat. The news continued reporting the day's events, including the passing of Glen Campbell. I stopped cutting for a moment and watched as a brief history of the musician's life was shared, including his very public battle with Alzheimer's. Mom struggled to rise from her chair, grunting and mumbling. I turned my focus back to Mom.

Me: What do you need, Ma?

MIL: I want…I want (stopping and sighing loudly) I want…YOU KNOW (pointing to the cutting board).

Me: The beets aren't cooked yet, Ma…they aren't very goo…

MIL: I haven't (her voice escalating) eaten ALL DAY (humph)!

Me: Mom (pausing and proceeding with caution), Fred said you both had dinner an hour ago. Would you…

MIL: I DID NOT EAT!!! YOOOUUU don't know when I ATE!

Me: Mom? (putting the knife down and approaching her slowly) Mom?

MIL: WWWWHAT? How the hell do you know when I ate?!

My heart started to beat a little faster. I truly hated when we got to this place, it often required that quick pep talk in my head. *This isn't the woman you love, find your patience, it is not your fault, she is confused and scared.* I took a deep breath and placed my hand gently on her arm. I had learned that she reacted well to a tender touch and gentle, genuine expressions of love. With this I started to guide her back to her chair.

Me: Mom? Would you like me to make a small snack?

MIL: NOOO! (humph!)

Mom's eyes were still a little wild as I stroked her arm and flashed a warm smile.

MIL: No (quietly). No…

I heard the gravel in the driveway announcing Joe's arrival. She didn't seem to lash out at him like she did with me. It was a relief to know he was here.

Me: Joe's here.

MIL: Who?

Me: Joe, your baby boy.

MIL: Oh…

I could see Joe through the window, stepping out of the truck. I gave him a wave as Mom craned her neck, looking confused. I leaned down and kissed her forehead, she closed her eyes and smiled softly. I paused over her for a moment, then returned to the kitchen to work on the beets. I heard Joe's heavy boots hit the first stair.

Joe: (calling up the staircase) Hey, Ma!
MIL: Hi! (straining over her shoulder to see him and smiling widely)

Joe reached the top of the stairs and tossed me a smile. He walked across the floor, and with a few long strides reached Mom's chair. She was still smiling and watching him lovingly as he leaned down and kissed her. He turned and crossed the room and met me at the sink, as he placed a soft kiss on my lips, he stepped back and half smiled.

Joe: How's she doing?
Me: Well, we're a little calmer now. She had a little outburst about dinner.

Joe looked at his feet, I kissed his cheek. He understood she could be difficult. I tried not to share how mean spirited she could get, but after twenty-seven years of marriage he could read me like a book.

Me: I'm going to finish this up and then get her ready for her bath.
Joe: Thanks.

Joe crossed the room to sit next to Mom. She looked up at him and politely smiled.

I finished the beets and washed up the dishes. Before I headed to the bedroom, I stopped by Mom's chair to let her know her bath was next. I'm met with an inquisitive look.

Me: Ma? I'm going to get your bath ready; I'll be back for your teeth in a minute.
MIL: (sigh) Okay.

I set up the bath and went back into the family room to fetch Mom's teeth. After putting those to soak, I went and told Mom we were ready. I walked with her to the bedroom and entered the bathroom to turn on the shower.

We did our dance. I repeated over and over, "It's just bath night," "No, you need clean clothes, those are dirty ones," "Yes, you can use the toilet again if you need to." I listened to her sigh at every task and watched her try to keep her patience.

Then came our saving grace.

Me: Mom? Let's brush your hair out, come here and sit on the bed.
MIL: Okay...you gonna...ummm...gonna get to me okay? I mean...if I sit there? How you...umm...how...you...
Me: Yep, you sit. I'll be fine, we're old pros at this.

I climbed up on the bed next to her and tucked my legs under me. I rested my hand on the top of her head and tenderly pulled the comb through her hair. Her eyes were closed and she was wearing a slight smile. Her hair is thin. I could comb it in its entirety in mere seconds. Instead, I continue...

Me: Mom?
MIL: Hhhhmmmm?
Me: Does that feel good?
MIL: Sure does...

I continued slowly stroking the comb through her hair, she was so peaceful while I did this simple act. I knew it brought a sense of calm over her, but selfishly I did it for me, too. The opportunities for us to have these quiet, untroubled, comforting moments were far and few between.

Me: (giving her shoulder a quick squeeze) How's that Ma?
MIL: Goooood...you're so good to me, what do I owe you?
Me: (surprised) Owe me?
MIL: Yea, what's this gonna cost me?
Me: Ummmm...(smiling and looking right into her eyes). It's gonna cost you a hug and a kiss!

Mom reached up so quickly and wrapped her arms around me that she startled me for a moment. I slowly pulled back a bit.

MIL: Wait!

Mom kissed my check. A wave of love washed over me so quickly that I had to fight back a tear.

MIL: (laughing) That's cheap! I guess you'll be back every day!

Mom's eyes danced, there she was. I cherished those fleeting moments when I had her again.

Me: (laughing) You made a funny, Ma!
MIL: Hmmmm?
Me: (pausing and look deep into her eyes) I love you.
MIL: I love you, too (smiling).

We walked back to the family room where Joe had nodded off in the chair.

MIL: Oh, I was going to sit there (looking at Joe in her chair).
Me: He'll move.
MIL: No, let him sit.

Mom sat in Fred's chair and I pulled a kitchen chair up next to Mom's chair. Joe lifted his head from his slumber and smiled as he looked up at me. A new dance began. Mom asked how the kids were, I explained that Ashley was in Massachusetts now and Joey still lived at home. Mom was surprised each time I answered.

In the background, *Entertainment Tonight* was on, another story about Glen Campbell was running. I paused mid-sentence to watch part of an interview with Glen and his wife Kim. The interviewer was saying, "I understand there are good days and there are bad days. What's today?" Kim smiled and said, "Today...today is a good day!" She stroked Glen's hair and smiled.

I looked back at Mom as Glen Campbell's last song began to play through the speakers of the television, "I'm not going to miss you..."

MIL: How are your kids?
Me: Good Ma, Ashley is in Massachusetts and Jo...
MIL: No Kidding! Massachusetts?!

Well...today...today, for the cost of a hug and kiss, was a good day...

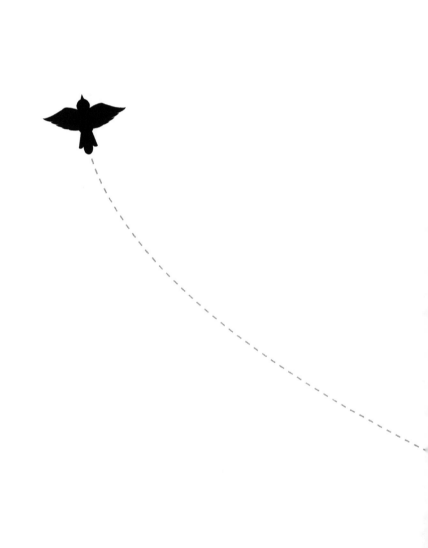

II

Challenging Times

Comprehending a New Normal

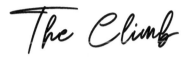

The Climb

September 2017

I'd like to paint you a picture.

Imagine flying like a strong eagle over a beautifully serene beach. The warm sun on your face, the waves gently slapping the soft sand, it is so peaceful and enjoyable you could glide carefree for hours. The wind guides you gently away from the shoreline, as you rise effortlessly over the dunes with confidence and ease. You sweep through the marsh lands, pumping your wings and watching the tops of the grass gently lay to the side as you brush by.

On the other side of the marsh your feet land firmly on somewhat solid soil, it's a little muddy but firm. The gooey ground is unexpected, but still feels good on your toes. Your steps are confident and sure as you continue down a clearly marked pathway. As the path twists and turns, it enters a tree line. The trees and greenery become thicker, birds sing songs of guidance as you wander through, the sunlight is screened and becomes distorted by the heavier tree canopy. There are areas that cause you to stop, hesitate, and wonder if you've wandered off the path, but somehow you always find your way.

As you forge on, the path opens into flat, bright, open fields with warm breezes caressing your cheeks. You run your fingers through the wildflowers as you walk, smiling as the butterflies jump off and brush by your face. Occasionally a rock or stump trips you, but you quickly regain your balance.

Across the field you choose a dark thick wooded path. As you proceed you find the path starting to climb. Something makes you hesitate. Standing still you realize the carefree songs from the birds are replaced with an unsettling, occasional owl screech. The path below your feet is becoming increasingly rocky and slippery and your footing is no longer confident and steady. The light continues to dwindle.

The path becomes steeper and more rugged. Sharp shards of light create dark shadows through the thick greenery, blinding you temporarily if it catches your eyes just right. The path forces you to slow and evaluate each step, you take a short pause and glance over your shoulder. You look back on the terrain you have navigated, from the easy shoreline to this rugged, slippery, and rocky path. You almost can't believe how far you've come, how your path has changed. The maps don't show this, nothing has prepared you.

A glance up to where you are headed reveals an even more jagged, steep climb masked partially by incoming clouds. You can't see the top. You can barely see the next three feet. Stopping is not an option, so you carefully stretch your hand to the next rock, pulling yourself up while simultaneously searching for solid footing for your next step.

This is the journey with MIL, the journey of Alzheimer's, where the landscape is forever changing and you have no idea what is going to confront you next. The journey, at times, feels impossible until you look back on where you've been and realize that the path wasn't always easy, but you did it. There is a reason you can't see through the clouds quite yet.

You are navigating a steep, rocky, slippery, and difficult path; a path you figure out as you go.

I have heard it said that the best view comes after the hardest climb.

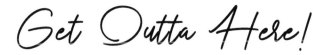

Get Outta Here!

Connecticut

September 2017

The gravel crackled under my tires as I pulled up the driveway. Fred was in the garage tinkering. I wondered what was in store for me that day as I climbed out of the driver's seat and called to Fred.

Me: Heya, Fred!

He looked up and nodded as I approached the open garage door. The garage was well organized, there was a place for everything, and everything was in its place. It was the space of a seasoned mechanic. Mom had always loved a man who could create with his hands and fix just about anything. While I may not have always agreed with Fred on what was best for Mom, I could see some of why she loved him so dearly.

Fred: Hey. She's up there (nodding toward the house).

I studied his face. It was there, I could see the veil of disappointment and frustration weighing on him. My guess was today was not a good day.
Me: How's she doing, Fred?

Fred shook his head, looked at his feet. He chewed a little harder on his toothpick then raised his eyes to me.

Fred: Well, ya know…
Me: I know, Fred. I heard the reunion picnic was tough.

Growing up, Joe had always considered his childhood friend Hans's mom a second mother. Bev had been everything Mom couldn't be for Joe. She had been home every day after school, she was a great cook who had dinner on the table promptly at 6:00 p.m. every night, she had the time to bake cookies and keep a tidy house. In a nutshell, Bev was June Cleaver, and Mom, on the other hand, often worked full time as well as doing the occasional side job to make ends meet. Raising five children on her own was not easy, or cheap. There were weeks at a time where she left for work as the sun rose and returned home well after bedtime.

Joe and I had seen Bev the day before and she had shared that Mom had had a few outbursts at the high school reunion. Bev told us Mom had become inconsolable and that she and Fred had to leave the picnic early. These reunions were special times, the pool of attendees was dwindling. My heart hurt for Fred. I looked up to the slider and saw Mom. She was sitting in her chair, leaning forward, elbows on her knees, staring intently through the window. I waved but she just continued to stare at me.

Fred: She sees us (shaking his head).
Me: Fred, I know she is getting belligerent, difficult, and sometimes a lot to handle. How many more outbursts are you dealing with?
Fred: Ya know, it's with her dad (nodding toward the window again, then looking at the floor). She yells that I'd better make sure I tell him…

The slider slammed open. Fred's head snapped up and an icy chill ran down my spine, despite the warm temperature of the early September afternoon.

MIL: (screaming) HEY! WHATCHA DOIN' THERE?!

I attempted to defuse the situation with a perky greeting.

Me: (waving and smiling) Hi, Mom!
MIL: (scowling) I said…whatcha doin'!?
Me: Just talking. I'll be right up.

Fred watched as Mom retreated through the slider and slammed it hard. I looked at Fred and sighed.

Fred: You better get up there.
Me: It's not just her being confused about her dad, is it?

The door slammed open again.

MIL: (voice escalating) Hey! I'm talkin' to YOU!
Me: Me, Mom? I'll be right up.
MIL: DON'T YOU DAAAAARE COME UP HERE!

I thought for a moment, *Maybe I won't!* Mom's eyes were wild, her nostrils were flared, and her lips were grimaced into a straight line.
Fred: You better…

The slider slammed again, this time so hard it popped back open.

Fred: (shaking his head) You better get up there.
Me: I'm going.

I made my way to the house, opened the door, and gently closed it behind me. I could hear Mom grumbling at the top of the stairs.

Me: (calling cautiously from the bottom of the stairs) Mom?
MIL: (screaming) GET OUTTA HERE!
Me: Mom (climbing the first four stairs)…Mom? It's…
MIL: (screaming) GET OUTTA HERE!

I took a deep breath and continued to climb. At the top step I paused and tried to assess what I was walking into. Mom was standing by her chair, her hands on her hips, and breathing heavy. She was clearly angry…and I thought maybe scared.

Me: Mom…(starting to cross the floor slowly).
MIL: GGGGGGEEET OUT OF HERE! (taking a step toward me).

99

Me: No, Mom…(approaching her and reaching for her arm) No, I'm here because I miss you, Mom.

MIL: (abruptly dropping into her chair) WHAT ARE YOU DOIN'?!… WHAT DO YOU WANT?!?!

Me: (sitting on a stool directly in front of Mom) Mom? Do you know who I am?

Mom was glaring directly at me, she raised her hand. I flinched, afraid for the first time ever that she might actually strike me. Instead, she pointed her finger at my face, just inches from my nose.

MIL: I know EXACTLY who you are and EXACTLY what you are up to!

Mom's face was red and had turned into an angry snarled mess. I suddenly realized what was going on and a lump rose in my throat.

Me: Mom? Do you think I was down there flirting with Fred, trying to take him from you?

MIL: NO!

She turned her head defiantly from me, her eyes darted back toward me. I thought, *If they were lasers I'd be fried right now.*

Me: Mom? I'm Lisa…I'm your…

MIL: I KNOW WHO YOU ARE…I KNOW WHAT YOU ARE UP TO!

I jolted my head back, her voice chilled me to the bone. I leaned forward and slowly, like I was approaching a cornered dog, reached my hand out and placed it on her knee.

Me: Mom?

She turned quickly in her seat, pulling away from my touch. I didn't move. I tried again. Slowly approaching her knee with my hand. My heart was racing as I realized I did not know the woman in front of me. This was uncharted territory.

Me: Mom? (my voice just above a whisper). I love you and I miss you. I'm here tonight to spend time with one of my favorite people in the entire world.

She turned her head slowly toward me, the dark, angry curtain started to lift and Mom's face began to soften. I thought I saw an opening to turn this around.

Me: Mom? Can I hold your hand?

Mom turned her hand over and allowed me to slide my hand into hers.

Me: Mom? I'm Lisa, and I've missed you so much. Can we spend some time together?
MIL: I...I...don't...ummm...don't know why I yelled.
Me: It's okay, Mom (starting to let my shoulders relax a little bit).
MIL: Why? I...I'm (tapping her head)...I'm not sure...(sighing) why? Why I yelled.
Me: Mom, you've been sick for a while (squeezing her hand and reaching my other hand across to her leg, giving it a gentle squeeze). See Mom, you may not feel sick, all of this (pointing up and down her body) is going along working fine, but this (tenderly stroking the top of her head), up here, there is something very sick. Your brain doesn't work like it should anymore, so you become confused and angry at times.
MIL: (starting to cry) But I don't (sniffling) mean to...
Me: I know, Mom, I know (stroking her hand). It's okay...

We sat for a few minutes in silence, Mom wiping tears, me squeezing and caressing her hand. I honestly didn't know what my next move should be.

MIL: I'm sorry I don't know...
Me: (raising my finger to her lips) Shhhh, shhhh, shhhh. Let's not think about that. Let's talk about our evening together. Guess what tonight is?
MIL: I don't know...
Me: (smiling and making my eyes dance) It's bath night!
MIL: What? Bath night...what?
Me: You know, Mom, when I scrub your back and such...

The stairs groaned as Fred made the climb. I wondered if he heard things calm down and was thinking the coast was clear. Well, at that moment it might have been, but it could all change faster than a dog could grab a bone.

MIL: Who's coming up the stairs?
Me: (softly) Fred. (Then attempting a cheerful greeting) Fred! How you doin?
Fred: Question is, how are you? (eyes wide and inquisitive).
MIL: What? (looking to me confused) Why?…What (eyebrows starting to knit).
Me: We're good, Fred, thanks.

Mom softened again. I leaned in and kissed her forehead. I paused and looked at her carefully. The tender and kind woman I adored and loved so deeply was back.

Me: Mom? I'm going to get us ready for your shower.
MIL: Oh, I'd like that…
Me: Yep! And a good back scrubbin'!

Mom smiled as I left the room to prepare her shower. I stopped in the hallway and peeked around the corner to find her intently watching Fred and rocking ever so slightly in her chair. I knew these outbursts were becoming more and more frequent. Mom was slipping away faster and faster, testing our limits. It took a lot of energy, self-control, and strength to not lose our patience, or lash back out at her.

I headed to the bathroom to get things ready, then returned for Mom.

Me: Mom?! Ready?
MIL: Where we goin'?
Me: It's bath time.
MIL: Oh, I like that…yes, let's go…
Me: That's my girl.
MIL: (stopping and smiling) You're my favorite…(tapping her head) favorite…
    oh, I don't know (giggling), you are just my favorite.

I hugged her and kissed her forehead.

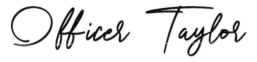

Officer Taylor

Connecticut

September 2017

The fourth stair tread squeaked as I stepped down, the squeak was simultaneous with my knee cracking as a yawn escaped my lips. I was tired, the kind of tired that makes your eyes burn, but equally invigorated. We were at the half-way point of our town's annual four-day Durham Fair, two more days to go. I paused at the staircase landing and stretched my back as I rounded the corner. In the kitchen, I heard the clinking of Joe's spoon as he stirred his coffee.

I leaned against the pantry door as he handed me my own steaming cup.

Joe: Good morning (leaning in for a quick kiss), how'd ya sleep?
Me: Like a rock.
Joe: You sure did! You were snoring to beat the band!
Me: (embarrassed despite twenty-seven years of sharing a bed) I did not!
Joe: (laughing) You did too!

I turned my back and playfully stomped away. As I entered the family room, I heard Joe slurp his coffee. I tossed a playful smile over my shoulder to find him already scrolling through his phone. This weekend and the weeks leading up to it could be all consuming. As Coordinator of Public Safety for the Durham Fair, Joe takes on an enormous responsibility—the health and safety of the fair's guests, volunteers, and vendors. He miraculously turned his team from a group of average volunteers, most with no public safety experience, into a force to be reckoned with. I'll never truly understand the pressure he is under during the weekend of the fair, but I strive to be the perfect supporter.

Me: Honey?
Joe: Hmm? (his eyes never leaving his phone)
Me: You think she's going to be okay tonight?
Joe: Who?
Me: Mom.
Joe: Hmmm? (clearly not listening, bringing his coffee cup to his lips again)

Joe's brother Scot and his wife Anna were picking Mom up from his brother Dave's that day. Fred works long hours parking cars at the firehouse for the fair each year. A few years ago we started sending Mom to Joe's brothers' houses over the weekend to enable Fred, Joe, and I to commit our time to our duties at the fair. However, Mom's recent changes and cognitive state had me worried ever since Dave picked her up that Friday morning.

Me: Joe!
Joe: (startled, looking up from his phone) What?!
Me: Did you hear me?
Joe: (eyes darting left to right) Ummmm…yes?
Me: (cocking an eyebrow at him) Oh yeah ? What did I say?

Joe gave me a sheepish grin as he placed his phone on the counter. I'm usually the one buried in my phone, only half listening. I explained to Joe that I was concerned about Mom staying in so many different locations in a short amount of time. We knew Alzheimer's patients didn't thrive with changes in scenery, especially overnight. Such changes would most often yield unpleasant outcomes. He attempted to put my mind at ease, but he wasn't completely successful.

The day went well. Saturday is always the longest and most intense day of the fair. It delivers our highest daily attendance and the biggest main stage act. Getting guests out safely and to their cars at the end of the night is always a balancing act, and honestly the volunteers start to get a little punchy. Afterall, they all have been stretched to the limits not only for the last three days, but for months.

When we arrived home around 11:30 p.m., Joe rested his head against the back of the driver's seat as he pushed the gear shift into park. A large satisfying sigh escaped his lips. He had just spent sixteen hours "steppin' and fetchin'" as well as overseeing the well-being of one hundred thousand guests, vendors, and volunteers.

Joe: Welp…another Saturday behind us.
Me: Another job well done by our fearless leader!
Joe: It's a team effort, I'm only as good as the people around me. Thank you…I couldn't do this without you.

I offered a weak smile and a shrug of thanks. Working public safety was the farthest thing from my chosen career. I was exhausted, there was nothing glamorous about the safety-orange shirt I wore, my nose was slightly sunburned, my feet were screaming, and I'd walked at least ten miles, half of them uphill. I opened the passenger-side door and hopped, or rather slid, out of the truck.

Me: Dibs on the shower first.
Joe: Go ahead, I need to spend some time with the girls.

Joe's "girls" were our dogs. As he bent down and nuzzled them, I climbed the stairs, listening to them whimper their love and admiration for him.

Joe found me in a deep, rewarding sleep when he crept into the bedroom. The sound of his shower briefly stirred me from my slumber, I glanced at the clock. It read 12:42 a.m., but the time barely registered in my brain as I fell quickly back into that beautiful, tranquil coma my body so desperately needed.

What seemed like minutes later, my phone chimed and I was jolted awake. Instinctively I knew if my phone rang in the middle of the night it was never good news. Groggily I smacked the nightstand trying to physically connect with my phone, the clock read 2:12 a.m. The bright screen announced the caller: FRED.

Me: Shit! Joe! (punching his arm, definitely harder than warranted) Fred? Hello Fred? What's the matter??
Fred: Well…we have a situation. Rosemary got lost.

Me: What?! (my voice hitting a deafening shrill)

Fred: The Suffield Police called me. They have Rosemary, here's the number of the officer you can call to give him Scot's address.

Joe was watching me with sheer panic in his eyes. I put the phone to my chest and told him to call Scot, that the Suffield Police have Mom. The panic faded as he immediately switched into first responder mode and picked up his phone to call his brother. I was literally shaking trying to write the phone number down, yet Joe was unshakable in his response. I read the number back to Fred and hung up without saying goodbye. Using every ounce of concentration I had, I started to dial the officer's number as I heard Joe connect with Scot.

Joe: Scot, where's Mom?...No...Fred says the police have her...I...I don't know. Just check...it'll be okay.

I watched Joe's face as my line rang. That switch in his head had flipped, he wasn't Mom's son right then, he was assessing an emergency.

Officer Taylor: Suffield PD, Officer Taylor speaking.

Me: (taking a deep breath to steady my voice) Officer Taylor this is Lisa Davenport, I am Rosemary Zieroth's daughter-in-law.

Officer Taylor: Good evening, Ma'am. I have Rosemary here with me.

Me: (voice cracking) Oh, thank God. Is she okay? Where...where...was she, Officer?

Joe shook my shoulder, pulling the phone away from his ear.

Joe: Scot sees the officer's car outside. He's going to meet him.

Officer Taylor: She's very disoriented, confused, otherwise she's...hold on please.

I wait as the line becomes muffled.

Joe: Does the officer see Scot?

Me: I don't know, he told me to hang on.

Joe: (talking into the phone) Scot, do you see the officer?...Taylor...yes...okay, good...yeah, then call me back.

Joe dropped the phone into the crumpled sheets. What in reality was only a moment or two felt like hours as I waited for Officer Taylor to return to the line.

Officer Taylor: Ms. Davenport? I have Scot Davenport here, your brother-in-law correct?
Me: Yes, oh my God, yes (choking back tears).
Officer Taylor: I'm going to release Rosemary to him. Have a nice evening, Ma'am.

The line disconnected. I looked at Joe and started to sob uncontrollably. He reached across the bed and gathered me in his arms.

Me: Call Scot back. WHAT happened?!?
Joe: Let him get Mom settled.
Me: How did she get LOST?!
Joe: Honey, I don't know…I…
Me: Don't they realize you have to WATCH her?

Anger was building in my chest. My voice was rising to an ear-piercing screech.

Joe: Stop, okay? Just. Stop.

I instantly felt like a child being scolded.

Me: Stop? (reacting mostly like a rotten teenager) Really? We ask for one weekend off and this happens?! I don't even want to talk to them, your family has no idea what we do, I'm done!

I flopped onto my side, turned my back on him, and pulled the covers tightly over my shoulder.

Me: (from my side of the bed) YOU call him and find out what happened!
Joe: He'll call me shortly (resting his hand on my shoulder). Honey?

I snapped my shoulder away from him and started to sob, an ugly, scary cry. The what-if's played out in my head and I cried harder. Joe's phone rang and he got out of bed and walked down the hallway out of my earshot. My little temper tantrum subsided and I strained to listen to what Joe was saying.

Joe: She is…no…no…no…it is not your fault. It's hard to guess what she's going to do. I just thank God she picked up Fred's bag. . .. How's Anna? No, tell her she didn't do anything wrong. We've been dealing with a lot. We'll catch up after the fair. Try to get some rest. . . Yeah, I will…good night.

The door creaked open as Joe turned off the hall light. He felt his way around in complete darkness and lowered himself into the bed. I rolled over and wrapped my arms around his chest, pulling him as close to my body as I could. He was strong and solid, a place of safety and assurance. I selfishly allowed myself to break down again. As I did, he turned his body into mine, pulling me equally as close. He brushed my tear-soaked hair away from my face, then wiped any remaining tears with his thumb.

He started to whisper, telling me the turn of events that led to the distressing call.

Mom had packed her bag, actually Fred's bag, which thankfully had his last name and "Durham Volunteer Fire Company" embroidered across the side. She had walked down the staircase, out the front door of Scot and Anna's house, and proceeded down their street. She walked past about two houses and crossed the street. She then walked up to the front door of the house across the street and started banging on the front door, yelling for Fred. There were no exterior lights on at the house, it was a miracle she didn't fall and hurt herself. The neighbors didn't know Mom was Scot's mother, but did realize she was confused and distraught, so they called the police. When Officer Taylor arrived, Mom couldn't tell him her name, her address, where she was, or even what year it was. The officer took a shot and called Durham Fire's Chief of Service who was able to share Fred's phone number. That's when Fred called. He had apparently tried to call Joe first, but it went right to voicemail. Joe apologized to me for having to take the call. I pulled my head back, actually offended.

Me: What are you apologizing for?!
Joe: She's *my* mom.

Me: I'm sorry I flew off the handle. I was scared, and I had a gut feeling about this weekend. You know how I hate it when my gut is right.

Joe: We need to make some changes.

Me: Yep, we do.

Joe: Tomorrow we start by ordering an ID bracelet.

Managing Expectations

Connecticut

November 2017

It was the Sunday morning before Thanksgiving. I stood in my kitchen in complete panic mode, I was showing shades of Ruth, Amy's mom from *Bad Mom's Christmas*. Joe had just reported that the thirty-six-pound turkey that was supposed to be defrosting in the carriage house fridge for the past four days was still frozen solid. There was some hyperventilating and shrill speaking when Joe, the always practical, sane, and reasonable person in our marriage, looked across the kitchen.

Joe: Honey, breathe. It's going to be fine. We'll buy a smaller turkey. We can't even fit this thirty-six-pound mother in the roaster!
Me: You don't understand, my sister raised it. I *have* to cook it!

My sister Debbie and her family had decided to raise turkeys early last year. She had proudly presented me with this turkey and was so excited for it to be used for our family Thanksgiving. I feared she would be devastated if it didn't work out.

Joe: Stop it. Let's save it for the firehouse or another occasion. I'm not even home to help you the day before. We'll buy a fresh one today. I'm sure Stew Leonard's has some we can pick up.
Me: (wringing my hands) I don't know I need to let Debbie know first.

Joe: Oh my God, Lisa! Get a grip! It's a turkey (grabbing his keys). C'mon, I'm buying you breakfast.

Reluctantly I pulled on my coat and walked to the car. As we drove, Joe took my hand and stroked the top of my thumb. I thought for a moment, *How does he do that?* I was beginning to relax. I could actually feel the stress leaving my shoulders. I watched him drive for a bit, then relaxed against the car seat, and smiled. The moment was broken with a startling ring through the speakers of my car. I glanced at the console to see Fred's name as the incoming call. Concerned I looked at Joe and pressed accept.

Me: Hi, Fred!
Fred: Well, hello there.
Me: All okay, Fred?
Fred: Well, I have a situation.
Me: Okay…Have you made plans to head back to Florida?
Fred: No, I have way too much going on.
Me: Ummmm, you need something?
Fred: Yeah, I have Fire Police training Monday night and Tuesday Night. Ya know I have Firehouse, and I'm thinking we're probably gonna stay in for Thanksgiving…so…
Me: So, you need someone for Monday night and Tuesday Night?
Fred: Yeah…I need to leave by quarter of six Monday…and usual time Tuesday…

Instantly my head began to spin. My to-do list was extensive.

Me: Okay, Fred. We'll work it out (looking at Joe still driving). I'll come by tomorrow and shower Mom, and I'll see if Dave might be able to do Tuesday. I've got a lot on my plate this week with Thanksgiving dinner. Speaking of which, what would you like to do for Thanksgiving? We'd love to have you join us!

I hoped my not-so-subtle hint might sway Fred to change his mind about staying in for the holiday.

Fred: Yeah, well, I need to leave at 5:45 for Fire Police Training Monday…

Me: Yes, I'll be there Fred, don't worry.

Fred: I don't know about Thanksgiving...maybe just us at home.

Me: Well, let me know what you decide. We'd love to have you at the house, or, ummm...I guess...umm...I could make you a separate dinner and bring it over.

I placed my palm to my forehead and shook my head. Joe looked at me like I'd totally lost my mind. I thought maybe I had.

Fred: Yeah, probably that...we'll just stay in...

Me: (looking at Joe in complete panic mode again) Ummmmm, well how about you think about it?

Fred: Okay, well, I'll see you tomorrow, 5:45. I need to leave by 5:45.

I hit end on the screen and Joe looked at me shaking his head.

Me: Do you think he needs to leave at 5:45? (sarcasm dripping in my voice).

Joe: You can't cook them dinner *and* make dinner for our twenty-plus guests. Be real!

Me: What am I gonna do? I can't leave them without Thanksgiving dinner!

Joe: No, we can't, but she's *my* Mom and...

Me: Let's see...

I felt this horrible pull. I couldn't leave Mom and Fred without Thanksgiving dinner, but realistically Joe was right. How did I think I could do both? I didn't even have enough ovens! Joe kept me centered throughout the day. We had breakfast out, shopped for dinner, secured another turkey, and found ourselves literally laughing like schoolchildren by the time we got home.

As Joe parked the car, he said he'd unload the groceries.

Joe: Go ahead in and make sure there's room for the turkey in the fridge.

Me: Okay, I'll take a few bags, too.

Joe: Honey, I've thought about it, Fred's gonna have to bring Mom for dinner. I want to see her and...well you just can't do anymore.

I looked at him and thought, *I'd walk over hot coals if you needed me to,* yet I felt an enormous weight begin to lift off my shoulders. I climbed the back stairs thinking about my next hurdle: how to break the news to my sister that we'd be eating a Stew Leonard's turkey this week, not hers!

The following morning, I was immersed in my work with my team at the studio when my cell phone alerted me I'd missed a call from Fred. Ever since the Durham Fair weekend, I'd been a little skittish about calls from Fred, so I immediately return the call.

Me: Fred? Everything okay?
Fred: Oh, yeah. I just wanted to make sure someone would be here tonight.
    You know, I gotta leave by quarter to six.
Me: (rolling my eyes) Yep, I'll be there Fred.

Does he think I don't listen to him? I thought as I took a deep breath. Then I reminded myself of all the things he did for Mom.

Fred: Well, what do you think you're gonna do for dinner?
Me: Tonight for Mom?
Fred: Yeah, well they give us sandwiches and such…
Me: Ummm, okay. Well our plan was that I'd come by at 5:40, shower Mom
    and such. Then when Joe gets out of work, he'll come by and sit with her
    for the night. Ya know what? I'll ask Joe to pick up dinner on his way over
    from the firehouse.
Fred: That'd be good, and, oh yeah, I think we'll just stay in for Thanksgiving.

I felt the muscles in my shoulders tightening. I was thinking that my detailed schedule just got blown to Mars. How was I now going to fix an additional meal on Thanksgiving *and* make the perfect dinner for my family? Seriously this *is* how I think.

Me: Okay, Fred…I know Joe was pretty excited about sharing the holiday with
    Mom and you at our house.
Fred: I don't know…
Me: (reminding myself this wasn't my battle) You can discuss this tonight
    with Joe.

Fred: Sounds good…see you later.

Me: Yep, see you soon.

I hung up the phone, it was 3:00 p.m., I texted Joe to call me when he could, and the phone rang in a matter of minutes.

Me: Hello?

Joe: Hello, Sweetheart…whadya need?

Me: We need dinner for Mom.

Joe: Huh?

Me: Fred's gonna be eating with the Fire Police tonight. We need to do dinner for Mom. Can you pick up something on your way home?

Joe: Yeah, I got it.

Me: Love you.

Joe: Love you too. Thank you.

Me: See you later.

About an hour later, reality checked in and I remembered someone needed to let the dogs out if I was going straight to Fred's. I texted Joey, with a cc to Joe, asking if he could help. Joe immediately texted back reminding me that Joey was helping his girlfriend Emily's grandmother move and probably wouldn't have time.

At 5:35 p.m., I left my studio to head to Fred's. As I pulled out of the parking lot, I realized I hadn't heard back from Joey, which meant he was probably not stopping home to feed the dogs! I called him to double check, and he confirmed he was not going home. I decided I needed to get to Fred's because he had to leave at 5:45! The dogs, poor pups, well they'd have to wait until Joe got out of work and could swing by the house. I sent him a quick text to make sure he remembered to do so.

I pulled up to the house, parked, and entered the side door. I squared up my shoulders and put a smile on my face.

Me: (in an upbeat, sing-song voice) Hellllllloooo?!

Fred: We're up here!

Me: (chuckling) Of course you are!

MIL: Helllllloooooo?

I stop two steps into my climb up the stairs, shocked. She sounds so upbeat!

Me: Heya, Ma!
MIL: Heya, back at ya!

I could hear her smile in her voice. I quickened my step and arrived at the top of the stairs to see her looking over her shoulder at me.

MIL: Hi! How are ya?!
Me: I got no complaints!
MIL: Pppssshhh, you always say that.

Was this Mom? I couldn't believe she was so coherent. Fred and I made our typical small talk, he told me about an accident in town that afternoon, and then headed out to his meeting.

I looked at Mom and she smiled. She took my hand and stroked it gently. I looked at her and thought, *Wow she's almost Ma!*

Me: How ya doing tonight, Ma?
MIL: Aww, ya know…good…
Me: Yea, it seems like tonight's a good night!
MIL: Huh?
Me: (yawning) Nothing, Ma.
MIL: (yawning) Why you doin' that?
Me: (yawning) What?

I wiped the corners of my eyes, I'd yawned at least four times in a few minutes and now my eyes were watering.

MIL: (yawning) That!
Me: (giggling) They're catchy aren't they, these darn yawns (patting Mom's arm). I've gotta stop this yawning baloney and get your shower ready!
MIL: (yawning) Oh, okay!
Me: (yawning) Stop that! You're making me yawn!

MIL: You started it…

She was right, I had started it! I was enjoying her moment of clarity, and the exchange of yawns. As I set up her shower, I asked her to start undressing. I started to strip down as I assisted her. I checked the water temperature, decided it was an agreeable temperature, then directed her into the shower. I stepped in behind her and she looked at me.

MIL: I think I need these off (sliding her now shower-soaked glasses off her nose).
Me: Oh, yeah, I guess so!

I giggled a little and Mom looked up at me, shaking her head. Showering Mom now required me stripping down to my bra and underwear and getting into the shower with her. It was the only way I could ensure she got herself clean and didn't slip and fall.

MIL: Ummm, hey you better get rid of yours too.

I tapped my face and realized I was still wearing my own glasses. I started to laugh. Mom joined and the laughter became one of those belly laughs that, if you're not careful, will take you to your knees.

We finally got ourselves under control, finished our shower, and got dressed. I directed her to the family room where the wood stove would keep us warm. I got her settled in her chair and returned to the bathroom to tidy up.

When I returned, I found Mom sitting in her recliner, staring off into space.

Me: Hey, Beautiful!
MIL: (jumping, startled) Hey!
Me: Sorry, didn't mean to scare ya!
MIL: Well don't scream when you enter a room!
Me: I'll remember that!
MIL: Humph . . you should.

I smiled and stroked her cheek. I gingerly started combing her hair. The knots were getting worse and worse each time I showered her. I made a mental note to pick up a detangler like I used when Ashley was young. I heard the door close downstairs as Joe entered the house.

MIL: Okay, he's here…
Me: He? That's Joe, Ma.
MIL: Joe?
Me: Yes. Fred's at a fire meeting.
MIL: Oh…

Joe walked up the stairs. He handed out his hugs and kisses then explained that Joey had reached out to his friend Frank to take care of the dogs to save us time. As I continued to work on the rats' nest in Mom's hair, I asked about dinner.

Joe: Well, I thought if I went out after checking on the dogs I wouldn't be back here until after 7:30. Finish Mom's hair and I'll take us to Cozy Corner.

Cozy Corner was right around the corner in town and was always a good choice in a pinch.

Me: (looking down at Mom) Okay, she's been good tonight.

I finished up Mom's hair; it was so thin that it dried almost instantly. As I picked up the towel and comb, I shared with her that I'd bring a detangler next time. Saying it out loud made the odds of me remembering much better! Then I told her we were going to dinner.

MIL: (grumph) Okay…

She struggled to get out of the chair. As we walked down the stairs, every step was an effort. To keep her spirits up, I talked as I walked her down the stairs.

Me: Come on, Beautiful!
MIL: Mhmmmmm…
Me: Whatd'ya mean? You're taking these stairs like a rock star!
MIL: Humph…

As we arrived at the restaurant, I helped her into her seat. Her zipper got stuck in her coat, and I reached over to help her.

MIL: (sighing heavily) I can do it ya know, I'm not a baby! (her voice rising with every syllable)
Me: (dejected) I know.
MIL: I got it. Thank you (with a slight sharpness in her tone).

I watched her struggle, with no success, to open the coat.

Me: Here (leaning in to open the coat).
MIL: Oh…

Dinner got off to a rocky start. When our salads came, Mom attempted to salt hers. Joe gently explained that she shouldn't have the salt. She became annoyed that Joe took the salt from her, even scowled at him. It became a little dicier when we both reacted to her next feat, which was to pour her O'Doul's over her salad.

Joe and Me: Eeeeek! Ech easy!
MIL: WHAT?!
Me: (looking around the restaurant to see who's taken notice) It's okay, Ma.
Joe: Ma, that's your beer. You don't put that on your salad.
MIL: I *know* that! I'm not stupid! I know how to drink beer!

I nudged Joe and discreetly pointed to the chicken on Mom's plate. We were going to have to cut it for her.

Joe: Can I cut the chicken for you, Ma?
MIL: No! I *got* it (glaring up at Joe).

I looked at Joe, it broke my heart to see him watch her like this.

Me: Mom, I gotta tell Joe what I did today in the shower.
MIL: What?!

While she didn't soften, she was looking at me rather inquisitively. I took that as a sign to keep going.

Me: Well, Beautiful, if you remember, you considered firing me today because I forgot to take off your glasses before you got in the shower…and honestly, I forgot mine too!
MIL: (laughing) Oh yes! (laughing again).

I watched her, thinking if I continued this play we might be able to get through dinner unscathed. At that time, she could switch from one emotion to another so easily.

Handling her moods often made me feel like I was crossing an icy pond. I placed my foot carefully, taking each step with caution. There was confidence in my step when I didn't hear the ice creak or pop, and an overwhelming sense of anxiety and restlessness when it did. The slightest sign of danger had me quickly looking to the shore for safety.

Thankfully, we finished our meal with minimal issues. As we left the restaurant, I watched Joe guide his mom through the door. I wish the woman who was at the house when I arrived was here for him now. She grumbled about the cold as she slumped into the front seat.

We drove in silence back to the house.

Me: Honey, why don't I stay with Mom until Fred comes back?
Joe: No, I'll stay.

I looked up at him and smiled weakly. He quietly directed Mom to the stairs. As he held her elbow, guiding her gently, I turned the handle of the door to leave the icy pond. Safety and freedom were in my sights, I should have been thrilled, yet guilt washed over me.

The Black Eye

Connecticut

December 2017

The snow began to fall as I sat at the conference room table prepping for a Saturday morning conference call. To my right, on a scrap piece of paper, was my to-do list. I was flying out that week and I wanted to make sure I covered all my bases before I left.

- Studio: Pack files, draw up and send plans for tile and flooring, and follow up notes to conference call
- Stop to see Mom and Dad
- Shower MIL, bring conditioner
- Buy groceries
- Decorate tree
- Christmas list, order Hess trucks
- Laundry

I sighed deeply, thinking I'd need to be a wizard to get all that done before the snow piled up. I texted my mom, telling her I planned to swing by for a visit around 11:00 a.m. I hadn't seen my parents since Thanksgiving and a wave of guilt flowed through my chest.

The morning progressed, and, as it often happens, my time at the studio was taking longer than expected. As the snow piled up outside my window,

I realized it was already 11:30 a.m. I texted my mom again, saying I'd be leaving shortly. Her response was to not worry, that we could catch up when I returned from Florida. I looked at the snow, looked at the time, and felt that guilty surge return.

"I'll Be Home for Christmas" banged out through the speakers in my office. I checked in with Joe, who had been home sick for a few days, and told him I needed to see my parents and that I'd be later than 12:30 p.m. for his mom's shower. He said to take my time, she wasn't going anywhere in the snow. I asked him how he was feeling before hanging up. I mentally returned to my list and crossed off the grocery store, Joe would need to do that Monday, and another gush of guilt rushed in.

Christmas carols filled my car as I drove to my parents' house. The ride was incredibly peaceful. Snow has a way of deadening sound, and often makes me feel as if my head is resting in a luxurious down pillow. The tranquility was good for the soul, even though it was coupled with the cold. I rounded the corner to my parents' road as Jennifer Nettles sang, "Please celebrate me home." I shook my head, looked to the heavens, and chuckled a bit.

My parents are amazing, the guilt I felt for not spending time with them was self-inflicted. Our visit was carefree, filled with fresh baked breads in a judgment-free zone. They truly know how to "celebrate me home." I left my childhood home more relaxed. I started the car and called Joe.

Me: Hey, I'm leaving Mommy and Daddy's. I'm stopping home for the conditioner.
Joe: (coughing) I'll take a ride with you.
Me: Honey, it's fine, you stay home.
Joe: (sounding like a frog) I need to see her. I've been on antibiotics for three days. I'll keep my distance.
Me: See you soon.

The phone disconnected, my mood was changing, Joe joining me to take care of Mom always made the visits more enjoyable. On good days we all fed off each other's good spirits, on bad days Joe and I had each other to lean on. I didn't know what the day would deliver, but I wouldn't be alone to receive it.

The snow piled up on the roads as we made our way to Mom and Fred's house. Again I found peace in the fresh fallen snow as I watched the landscape change beautifully before my eyes. Joe interrupted my thoughts.

Joe: Hess trucks are all set for the boys. I got three, that's right, right?
Me: (crossing them off my mental list) Oh, great! Yes that's fine. Ummmmm…
Joe: What?
Me: It's already after 2:00, I don't think I'm getting to the grocery store (guilt rolling in).
Joe: We're fine, I can go tomorrow.
Me: I know, but…
Joe: Stop it.

Joe put the truck in park in Fred's driveway. I slid out of the truck, my feet landing in the snow with a soft crunch. Joe opened the door and called out our arrival. As we climbed the stairs, I saw the piles of dust and sighed. I added another thing to the to-do list in my head, time to clean this place.

We got to the top of the stairs. Mom was in her chair, watching the snow through the window. Joe walked behind her to pet the cat and headed directly across the room to hang his coat on the kitchen chair. I turned the corner and approached Mom. When I saw her, I sucked in a quick breath. The entire right side of her face was black and blue. Experience told me I needed to remain calm, an outburst would just startle and upset her. I approached her carefully and squatted down in front of her chair.

Me: Hi, Ma.
MIL: Hello.
Me: (stroking her hand) Ma, you okay?
MIL: Yeah, why?
Fred: (turning from the wood stove) Oh, yeah, she took a spill.
Me: (looking across the room to Joe) Mom, does your face hurt?

Concern flashed across Joe's face as he watched me. When he approached his mom, I saw his face fall.

Joe: Mom?

MIL: What?

Joe: (reaching up and gently tilting her head toward him) Does your face hurt? (never taking his eyes off Mom) Fred, when did this happen?

Fred: When you were gone. I checked her, she's fine.

A wave of guilt so strong washed over me that I had to fight back tears.

Me: When Fred?

Fred: Earlier in the week.

Me: When we were in Maine?

Fred: I guess that's where you were.

Joe started to examine Mom's face, pressing here and there and asking if some spots hurt more than others, if she could see okay. He'd flipped his internal switch and gone clinical, which I was thankful for. I, on the other hand, don't have that defense mechanism. Joe and I had escaped over the weekend for our wedding anniversary, my cousin Mike and his wife Donna had joined us, celebrating their own anniversary. The trip was supposed to be a good reset button for us, and it was, although now I was regretting the time away. If we had been home, would this have happened? My head was spinning with what-ifs, mixed with a healthy dose of anger that Fred hadn't contacted us.

Joe: Fred, when earlier this week did this happen?

Fred: Ummm…Monday. Yeah, she was arguing with me about getting in the shower. I told her to wait for me. She didn't. She was hollerin' and tried to get into the shower herself. She slipped and hit her head on the toilet paper holder and banged up her back too.

Joe: Fred (clearly trying to keep his voice calm and not judgmental), I've told you we have to know immediately if she takes a fall like this. She's on Plav…

Fred: (dismissively) You…you were gone, I watched her.

Joe: (looking at the floor and shaking his head) With the medication she's on, she needs to be seen right away; she could have had brain bleed.

Fred's tone is infuriating, I was struggling to keep my composure and not fly off the rails and lash out. Joe asked Mom to stand up so he could see her back.

I helped her stand, which was a struggle. I slid her shirt up and held my breath. The bruise covered a good part of her right side. Joe let out a deep sigh.

Joe: Mom, can you take a deep breath?

MIL: Yeah...

Joe: Could you do that for me?

MIL: (sucking in a long breath) Like that?

Joe: Yep (gently pressing around the bruised area). Does this hurt?

MIL: Little...ppshhhhh...

Joe: Okay, let's sit you back down.

MIL: (wincing as she starts to sit) Oh, oh that...(turning and putting more weight on her left foot, easing her way back into the chair). Phew...that's better (settling back into her chair).

Joe: Fred, we're going to need to get someone to come in and help her shower, a home health...

Fred: (cutting Joe off) Well, ya know we have that other shower. I put her in there the other day, she hates it, she yells and fights me.

Joe: She can't be alone to shower, and Lisa can't be here every other day to shower her.

Fred: She does okay.

Joe: I think we need to...

Fred: I get her in. She argues, but I get her in.

This is how it went; Fred was in his own state of denial. Mom needed more help, and he wouldn't admit it. It was becoming more and more contentious between Fred and us. He had taken to telling his friends at the firehouse how difficult we were and more. The negativity was difficult to hear and accept.

Me: Fred, can I use that shower today? I'm worried she can't step over the tub in your bathroom.

Fred: Yeah, that's fine...

He grunted and wore a scowl as he looked at me and Mom. I couldn't imagine what he was going through, I knew first-hand that Mom could be difficult. Still, the only help Fred would accept was us, and there were just not enough hours in a day to care for Mom and live our lives. I turned and I looked at

Mom. She looked like she'd been through a battle. I had been sick the previous week so I hadn't showered her before our trip, I had just come for a short visit. As I assessed her, I could see her hair was matted and her teeth were in desperate need of attention. I could only imagine what other parts of her body needed attention.

I gently guided her into the shower. This shower was tight, but it didn't require me to strip down myself and get into the shower with her. I watched as she let the warm water pour over her head.

Me: Feels good huh, Ma?
MIL: Ummmm, yeah.
Me: Temperature okay?
MIL: Yeah.
Me: Wow, I got the temp right on the first shot! I'm getting pretty good at this!
MIL: Yeah, you're hired.

I poured the shampoo into my hand and gingerly started to wash her scalp. I could see now, with her hair wet, how far the bruise extended up her scalp.

Me: I'm not hurting you, am I?
MIL: No…you never do.
Me: Good.

As I massaged the shampoo into the back of her hair, I could feel the knots and wondered if I'd make headway with the conditioner. Mom asked, like she did during every shower, why I was so good to her. We did our dance—I told her it was because I love her, she said she loved me back, and around and around we went.

Settling Mom into her chair by the fire, I took to her rat's nest at the back of her head. I tenderly combed through her hair. The conditioner had helped, but it still took me quite some time to get the comb through her hair. As I did, I became lost in my own thoughts. My mind wandered to my own parents, it drifted to the visit we just had, how I had walked through the back door and been greeted with hugs and smiles. They are sharp, they are healthy, and I am so blessed.

The comb finally slid through Mom's hair smoothly. I craned my neck around to see her face as I did so. Her eyes were closed, and she was wearing a slight smile.

Me: Like that, Ma?
MIL: Ah yeah…

I continued to comb her hair. I glanced at Joe, I could see the stress in his face and my heart broke. I pulled the comb through her hair one more time and kissed the top of her head, making eye contact with Joe as I wink.

Me: There ya go, Beautiful!
MIL: Aww, thanks…
Me: (resting my hand on her shoulder and looking at Joe) Whadya say, Honey? Snow's comin' down pretty good. Think we should head out?
Joe: Yeah, probably should…
Me: Love you, Mom. I'll see you next weekend. I'm leaving for Florida on Tuesday.
MIL: Oh?
Joe: I'll be here Tuesday night with you, Mom.
MIL: You will? Why?
Joe: Fred goes to the firehouse.
MIL: Oh…Okay!

The short drive to our house was quiet. The radio played "Santa Claus is Coming to Town" as the wipers skipped across the windshield.

Me: Who was with Mom Tuesday while we were in Maine?
Joe: (raising his hand in dismissal) My brother.
Me: Shouldn't he have called?
Joe: I can't go there, it's…(shaking his head and glancing away).

We continued in silence, I battled with the guilt of not knowing Mom took the fall, the worry of what could have been, and being upset that we didn't get a call Tuesday. I realized that Joe and I understood the ramifications of such a fall, while others didn't, and I tried to keep things in perspective. Fred said she was okay and that was why we didn't get a call. Joe understood this too.

We knew we couldn't be upset that we didn't get a call, so what good would come from calling his brother and getting upset? In Scot's mind, Mom was okay, Fred had said so. Joe pulled the truck up to the sidewalk of the house.

Joe: Hop out.
Me: You going somewhere?
Joe: No, I just was dropping you closer to the door so you don't have to walk through all the snow.

I leaned over and kissed his cheek. The afternoon had taken a toll on him; he had to be consumed with his mom's well-being, still, he put me first. I reached for the door handle as Joe's hand landed on my shoulder.

Joe: Thank you…
Me: For what?
Joe: For everything you do for her.

I kissed his hand and looked up at his face. He looked so tired. I often struggled to understand what Joe was going through. It must have been difficult to watch his mother fade away. Did he question if he was doing right by her? I knew he felt alone in this journey with his mom. The burden of making decisions about his mom's care weighed almost solely upon him, the youngest of five. We were a team on this journey, yet I expect he carried some guilt about needing to rely on me so much. I often wished I could express to him that taking care of his mom was, in my eyes, an honor, not a burden. That's what love is.

Me: It's not a big deal…how about we find a movie and just hang out for a bit?
Joe: Sounds great.

We nestled into the sofa to watch *National Lampoon's Christmas Vacation*. Ten minutes after it started, we were both asleep. Sleep is a great escape, there's no guilt when your brain shuts down for a bit.

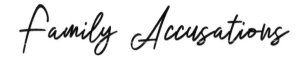

Family Accusations

Connecticut

December 2017

The house was quiet as my fingers flew across the keyboard. I sipped my coffee, reliving the previous night's discovery and running through the details in my head. My mind searched for the right words, the best way to share our night without being judgmental or unkind.

I read and reread my words and questioned if I should share the events of the previous evening with my Facebook followers. Mom's voice filled my head, "Don't stop, keep going…it may be the only way I can help others." I returned to a few previous posts and read the comments.

> *"This is a tug at the heart for all of you…Such a journey…I know it well. Blessings to you to share your day with her too… This whole short story is poignant! I send prayers…and pensive thoughts to you!"*

> *"Lisa, what you are doing is straight from your heart. You may get tired, but you will never ever have even one regret. Treasure the time."*

"Thx, it so good to know we're not alone in the journey."

"Thanks for once again capturing and documenting this difficult journey. We are on such parallel paths and have similar interactions."

"Lisa, you're amazing! My grandmother had this disease, the similarities you describe above are strikingly similar. I would give anything to have another day with her. She was such a kind, caring, charismatic, and amazing woman. Are you sure you're not a novelist? (ghostwriter?) Man, you sure can write and describe very vividly!"

"Wow. You two are the greatest. You only have one mom in life. I love these stories. Kinda reminds me almost of that movie, The Notebook. Seriously you oughta write a book. I know sometimes it's hard, but you guys have the patience and willpower. My mom has severe dementia and sometimes I catch myself asking her, "Do you remember?" She really doesn't recognize me anymore; she thinks I'm my older brother. It's hard sometimes but I get through it. I miss the old mom before this disease but at least she is still here. You guys are a great inspiration."

Staring at the computer screen, I heard Mom's voice again, "Help me help others." With a deep breath and a bit of courage, I copied and pasted the story into my feed. My cursor hovered over the blue "post" button. Why was I so hesitant? I reread the post again, and decided it was good. It was hard to share, but good. I hit "post," closed my laptop, and slid it onto the coffee table. The morning news reported icy conditions and cautioned drivers to take extra time for the morning commute. Our dog Izzy was sprawled across my feet, her heavy frame a welcome comfort. I leaned down and stroked her velvet soft ears and asked her if I had made the right decision. Then chuckled to myself, *Does a one-hundred-pound Rottweiler hold all the answers?* Izzy turned her head toward me and nestled it into my lap, her own sign of approval. With a gentle pat, I informed the ole wise dog I needed to get ready for my day.

I made it to the studio and finished a morning of meetings and conference calls. The microwave chirped, announcing my soup was warmed. My designer, Katie; design assistant, Sara; and studio manager, Laurie, were hard at work managing last-minute details for a holiday delivery. I thought I heard one of them chuckle when the microwave emitted its weak beep. We'd been fighting with the old, hand-me-down machine for the last few months. It was on its last leg and hardly warmed anything anymore.

Me: (passing the work counter) Whadya think? Will four minutes in that old battle box do the trick in warming my soup?

Katie: I don't know, my pasta took two rounds of three minutes!

Sara: Mine warmed in one shot…five minutes.

Me: (rolling my eyes) Well, what do we want for free?! Maybe Santa will bring LDD a new microwave!

Katie: (bouncing in her seat like a child) Please? We've all been such good girls! Right, Laurie?

Laurie: (laughing) We have been! Santa won't find us on the naughty list!

The microwave sent out a distressing chirp as laughter filled the room. My soup was lukewarm, but I decided it was good enough for me. I joined Katie and Sara at the work counter as Laurie pulled up a stool and unwrapped her sandwich. I watched my team chatting about the upcoming holidays, who was hosting, what cookies were being baked, and how much shopping was left to do. I loved the chemistry in the room, a wave of pride flowed over me, I had assembled a great team.

Sara: Lis, you must be excited about your family trip to Florida after Christmas!?

Me: (without any sign of enthusiasm) We are.

Katie: Huh? You don't sound like it!

Me: It was a rough night with Mom last night. Joe and I haven't talked about it, but I'm wondering if we should go.

Laurie: I read the post this morning. Is she okay?

Katie/Sara: (equally raising their voices in concern) What happened?!

I relived the previous night's discovery with the girls. I shared that, for the first time since starting *Life with MIL,* I wasn't sure I should share what had happened. Yet, in the end I remembered I had made a promise to Mom to keep telling the story. I only hope I wrote it without judgment and filled with gratitude and grace.

Laurie: I read the post. I think you told a story that had to be told. You weren't judgmental. I thought you and Joe had to be frightened to death when you saw her, and I wondered how you kept it together!

Me: Thanks, Laurie, I'm still not sure on this one.

Katie: (smiling, looking at her phone) Well, you've got quite the response. There are twenty-three comments! (her face falling) Oh no, I think you better read these.

Me: Shit…bad?

Katie: Well one? Go read them.

I left my half-eaten bowl of soup on the worktable and bolted to my office. My hands shook a bit as I logged into Facebook. I had forty-one notifications, almost all of them directed to that morning's post. I opened the post and started reading. The first dozen or so were positive, full of support, love, and understanding. Then I was jolted by a post from a family member of Fred's, and the firestorm it ignited.

A wave of heat rose from my chest and up over my face as I continued to read. She fired off allegations of abuse, neglect, and exploitation of her stepfather, all directed against Joe and me. Our community of followers of *Life with MIL* responded with their own bombs of retaliation. Her response was a rain of missiles that included threats to call the Department of Family Services, and the Connecticut State Police to report elder abuse.

Tears stung the backs of my eyes as I read. Joe had expressed some concern over the last few months about *Life with MIL*. Fred obviously didn't want the story told; I'm certain it was the reason he started spreading rumors and untruths about Joe and me through the volunteer firehouse and town. I had explained to him that a promise was a promise, and this was one I couldn't break. Now I was beginning to think I had made a serious mistake. The back of my throat hurt, I picked up the phone and dialed Joe.

Joe: Hello?

Me: Honey (my voice cracking as I sucked in a quick breath)…I'm sorry…

Joe: What? What are you talking about?

Me: I…I…(struggling to explain what was unfolding before my eyes) I think…I…

Joe: (clearly losing patience) What is going on?!

Me: *Life with MIL* (sniffling)…I posted this morning…

Joe: Oh, no (sighing deeply). What happened (his voice quiet yet laced with disappointment).

Me: I tried to…I really don't think I…I never meant…

Joe: Geez…can you just tell me what happened (his frustration clearly coming through the phone).

Me: (taking a deep breath) Karen is threatening to call the Department of Family Services and the state police. She is accusing us of neglect. She said we dumped Mom at Fred's and that we're taking advantage of him (tears welling up in my eyes, a quick hiccup escaping my throat). She…she says… we…we're using him to take care of our responsibility, which is abusive. She said Mom's become his financial burden while we live our lives with…

Joe: Okay, stop. Take the post down right now.

Me: I didn't mean…please don't be mad.

I quickly screen shot the comments then moved the cursor over the post and deleted it.

Me: It's done. I deleted it.

Joe: Okay, now let me do damage control. I've got some phone calls to make.

Me: I'm so sorry…I didn't think I was…

Joe: You know Fred has become difficult. You know he feels you're sharing too much, maybe you should have skipped this one.

The silence was deafening, the bite in his last comment hurt.

Me: (barely whispering) Sorry.

Joe: I'll call you in a bit.

The day became a rollercoaster of emotions. Dozens of private messages on Facebook flowed in, sharing support and encouragement. These were, thankfully, peppered between the calls from Joe with updates. He reached out to Fred's stepdaughter, Karen first and quickly realized he was not the person to reason with her. In anticipation of her making good on her threat to contact the state police, he reached out to our resident state trooper and good friend for guidance. He learned that while she can make the call and file a complaint, it would be difficult for it to be justified. We took some relief in that news, although we felt strongly that we needed to attempt to calm our accuser. Joe reached out to his brother Dave for help. Dave was more removed from the continual caretaking and could be a good mediator.

After work, I headed home, not sure what I was going to find when I got there. I cautiously opened the back door and stepped into the mudroom. Izzy rolled over and greeted me with a groan at my feet. Joe stood in the kitchen on the phone.

Joe: Yep…no…that isn't the…I know, yes, you're right.

He looked up and watched me as the conversation continued. I couldn't decipher who he was talking to.

Joe: I appreciate your help…maybe…yeah, bye.

He placed the phone on the counter and let out a deep sigh.

Me: (quietly) Who was that?
Joe: Dave.
Me: Oh.
Joe: He thinks he can defuse the situation.
Me: (relief flooding my voice) Oh, thank God.
Joe: Honey.
Me: Hmmmm?
Joe: You gotta stop.
Me: Stop?
Joe: Yes. Take a break.
Me: But (my lip quivering)…but I…I promised…
Joe: Just stop posting. Keep writing, but stop posting, especially right now.

I nodded my head, looking at the floor as a hot stream of tears flowed down my cheeks. It was never my intention to create division, hard feelings, or animosity as a result of posting these stories. It was always to help.

Joe: I've been thinking...
Me: (sniffling) About what?
Joe: Mom's too much for Fred. I think we need to move her.
Me: Where? (tears quickly stopping as I focus on his face)
Joe: If we get a full time caretaker, we can move her here.
Me: (my head starting to spin) Here? Where? She can barely do the stairs at
    Fred's. Our only spare bedroom is Ashley's...upstairs.
Joe: We could change the living room like we did for her when she rehabbed
    with us in 2001.
Me: I don't know...

Selfishly I remember the beautiful Thanksgiving we just had, how our house had been filled with family and friends. I thought about Joey and his friends who come and go easily. Would they still do that if Mom occupied the living room? Realistically, could we get a caretaker, and who would care for her at night? How would I travel between home and Florida with her living with us? My head spun.

Joe: I know it's a lot, but...

I shook my head and continued down that road of reasons why the arrangement wouldn't work, thinking, *How could I continue to run my business? Would we ever travel again? Where would I put my grandfather's sofa,* and *was I comfortable with a stranger in our home?* I stopped for a moment and looked up at Joe. His face was pleading with me.

Me: It is a lot. I know we did it when she was recovering from her fasciitis...

Mom had had a terrible case of necrotizing fasciitis in 2001. At the time we almost lost her to the horrific flesh-eating disease. She spent months in the hospital and rehab before we moved her into our home for six months to continue her rehabilitation.

Joe: We did (hope rising in his voice) and I was in paramedic school!
Me:…and she was of sound mind.
Joe:…and we had two young kids.
Me:…and Mom could be alone for hours on end by herself.
Joe: We'd get a companion.
Me: What about nights? We both work full time.…and when I travel, then
what?

His hand landed on my arm and he squeezed gently. I looked up into his face
and saw a man who loved his mother, a man who just wanted her to be in the
right place. He would have done anything for her. I watched his face, I saw the
sacrifices he had made for me over the years, how he had never really said no
to anything I had asked of him. How could I now say no to him?

Me: You're right. We can figure it out. Joey's old enough to help, and I'm sure
Ashley can help when she can come down. Maybe we can get some help
from your brothers too.

He quickly wrapped me in his arms, he held me tight as a soft sob escaped
his lips.

Joe: (burying his head in my shoulder) I'm sorry.
Me: Shhh (caressing his back). Sorry for what?
Joe: For yelling at you earlier on the phone.
Me: I should have asked you if I should post that first.
Joe: No, maybe the post had to happen. Maybe it's the beginning of our next
chapter. I know it won't be easy for Fred to give up on Mom. It'll take some
coaxing. It will give us some time to work on setting up help. Thank you.

I pulled away a bit and reached up to kiss his cheek. I searched his eyes, then
offered a gentle smile. I reassured myself that we could do this, and then silently
asked God for some help.

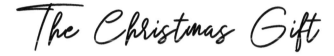

The Christmas Gift

Connecticut

Christmas Day 2017

The alarm buzzed at 5:30 a.m., pulling me from my very satisfying slumber. Joe reached across the bed and brushed the hair from my face.

Joe: Merry Christmas.
Me: Grumph…Merry Christmas.
Joe: (laughing) I'll make the coffee, you sleep.
Me: Hmmm…sounds good, but I gotta get up. I've got dinner to make for Fred and Mom.
Joe: You can sleep another half hour.
Me: Nah, I'm up. Plus, I'd like to spend a few minutes with you before you go to work.

I dragged myself from bed and threw on my robe. I walked past the closed doors of my babies' rooms. Stopping at the staircase, I rested my hand on the newel post and let out a soft sigh. There would be no jumping on their beds this morning. We broke tradition and celebrated our typical Christmas morning last night since Joe was working a twenty-four-hour shift today.

When I rounded the corner of the kitchen, Joe was pouring two cups of coffee. The light over the counter caught and reflected just right, revealing the silver that had filled much of his hair. I noticed his eyes were swollen from lack of

137

sleep. It had been a challenging month; we had to cancel a family trip due to the ever-changing condition of Mom. We fielded unwarranted accusations of neglect and lack of understanding of her current state, much of it sparked by that Facebook post about her fall. It was clear her illness was becoming too much for Fred, and she really couldn't make another trip to Florida. We needed to consider our next steps; would it be to move in with us as we had discussed again last week? We struggled to make the right choices on her behalf and seemed to always be second-guessing ourselves.

Joe: (handing me a steaming cup of liquid gold) So, what are you making for their dinner?

Me: (yawning) Turkey breast, stuffing, gravy…extra gravy, Fred said he needs extra (giggling), turnip…I must really like him because I *hate* the smell of turnip, mashed potatoes, sautéed green beans, and fresh apple pie.

Joe: (leaning in and kissing my forehead) Thank you.

Me: It's nothing, really (sipping the coffee). Oh, there's an extra chocolate pie for you to take to work, let me just whip the whipped cream.

Joe: Thanks, let's sit for a minute. You can make the whipped cream while I shower.

Izzy pushed between us as if she heard Joe's instructions. I watched her large frame wiggle as she led the way to the family room. That creature had really softened this Cruella de Vil's heart, partially because she had been so good with Mom over the years, she really had been her personal nursemaid. The dog groaned as she slid her face along the leather sofa and laid that big yet beautiful body right where Joe and I were about to sit.

Me: (dripping with sarcasm) It's okay, Izzy, we didn't want to sit on that sofa.

Joe: (chuckling) Don't listen to Mommy, Izz; you stay right where you are.

I climbed onto the sofa, carefully balancing my full cup of coffee as Joe squeezed onto the opposite end. I watched as he slid his feet under Izzy's back and he smiled, looking down at the dog. Moments like this were precious, our lives were so busy as we juggled crazy work schedules and caring for Mom, all the while questioning our choices. Joe leaned forward and turned on the local news. It was filled with Christmas music and a dose of good news, which was a welcome change.

Joe gently squeezed my leg, his way of telling me he was heading upstairs for his shower. I stretched and held my coffee cup up, batting my eyelashes. He shook his head and took the cup. I flipped through the channels on the television, stumbling upon *It's a Wonderful Life.* Joe leaned down over Izzy and handed me my coffee.

Joe: Here ya go, Princess.
Me: Thank you.

I settled back into the sofa, giving myself a few more moments with George and Mary.

> *"What is it you want Mary?" George Bailey was asking. "What do you want? You want the moon? Just say the word and I'll throw a lasso around it and pull it down. Hey. That's a pretty good idea. I'll give you the moon, Mary."*

I sipped my coffee as I heard the shower turn on upstairs, a smile crossed my lips. I turned off the television, wrangled my body off the sofa, careful not to disturb Izzy, and headed to the kitchen. I began to work my way around the kitchen, whipping the cream, unpacking the potatoes, and turning on some Christmas carols. As I packed up the chocolate pie for Joe, I heard him enter the kitchen, he looked refreshed and, frankly, so handsome in his uniform. He filled his coffee mug and pulled on his coat.

Joe: Thanks for the pie.
Me: Enjoy it!
Joe: Let me know how she is today, okay?
Me: Will do. Love you! Be safe.

He leaned down and kissed me. He took a step to pick up the pie and stopped. He turned toward me again and kissed my forehead. He rested his lips for a moment longer than usual and I could feel his love radiating through my body.

As I watched the back door close, I thought, *He'd lasso the moon for me.* We are an amazing team. We will get through this together.

The house slowly woke up. Ashley was first, which was a treat because she offered a much needed helping hand in the kitchen while she made her own pies for my parents' Christmas dinner. Her boyfriend Andrew made his way down wrapped in his blanket, then lastly, Joey. They opened their stockings filled with silly little toys and candies and lounged around watching Christmas movies.

Then it was time to head out. I packed up dinner and rounded up the kids.

Me: Come on, guys, I want to spend a few minutes with Grandma Z before we go to Mimi and Papa's.
Ashley: We're set.
Joey: I need to pick up Emily. Can I meet you at Mimi's?
Me: Yeah, that's fine. Maybe see Grandma this week?
Joey: Yep.

The fresh fallen snow created a Christmas card scene as we drove to Mom and Fred's. Fred had plowed the driveway, so our ride up was carefree and easy. Andrew and Ashley loaded up their arms with hot trays of food as I waved to Mom through the window. I pushed open the door and called up the stairs.

Me: Merry Christmas!!!!
MIL: Hello?
Me: (climbing the stairs) Hi Mom! Merry Christmas!!!
MIL: Well, hello…and Merry Christmas to you too?
Me: (chuckling) Yeah, it's Christmas, Ma. How are you?
MIL: Good…whadya got there?
Me: Ashley, Andrew, and Christmas dinner for you and Fred!
MIL: Oh really?!

Mom was smiling, her eyes seemed clear and her smile bright. She tilted her head and studied Ashley and Andrew for a moment. Fred was nowhere to be seen.

MIL: (pointing at Ashley) I know you...

Ashley: Yep, you do. I'm your granddaughter Ashley!

MIL: (slapping her hands to her thighs) I knew it! Yes, Ashley!

Ashley: Yep, we share a birthday and everything!

MIL: (studying Andrew) Oh?

Andrew: (waving) Hi!

MIL: Hi...do I know you?

Andrew: Yeah, I'm with her (smiling and pointing at Ashley).

Ashley: This is Andrew, Gram.... he took a road trip with us when we drove you back from Florida a few years ago.

MIL: (intently looking at Andrew) I...I think I remember that...

Ashley and Andrew reminisced about the trip, how fun it was, and how Ashley got lost in Washington DC. I watched Mom carefully as she was nodding, and I thought she was actually remembering the trip, or at least part of it. I heard the tractor coming up the driveway, I turned to watch a very bundled up Fred as he easily maneuvered the machine around my car and into the garage. I listened for the door to open downstairs and for Fred's feet to hit the first few stairs. I reminded myself to keep my patience, but, at the same time I am angry that he had left Mom alone.

Me: Well, there he is!

MIL: Who?

Me: Fred!

MIL: Oh, yeah.

Me: Merry Christmas, Fred!

Fred: Merry Christmas.

Me: Were you up doing Kate's driveway?

Fred: Yeah, and the garage.

Me: Boy, it's cold out there. You did a great job on the driveway here, made for an easy shmeasy ride.

Fred: Yeah, well...It's warm in here! Got the stove going good! Right, Rosemary?

MIL: Yep!

Me: Fred, I've got dinner over on the stove for ya. Want to see?

As Fred and I walked to the stove, I reminded myself it was Christmas. *Find the blessings today, Lisa; don't judge.* A sigh escaped my lips as I uncovered the dishes and showed Fred the feast we'd brought. When I peeled back the foil over the apple pie, a little steam rose off the top.

Fred: Apple pie, Rosemary will like that.
Me: You too, right?
Fred: Oh, yeah!
Me: (crinkling my nose) There's turnip, too!
Fred: Yeah, good, I like that.

I looked at Fred and thought this was the least I could do for him this Christmas. I was very grateful for all he had done for Mom. I felt an internal tug as Fred busied himself in the kitchen.

Fred: Well, we won't be eating for a bit...
Me: (feeling that tug) Fred, do you need something?
Fred: No, we're good?
Me: You sure?
Fred: No, we're gonna watch some TV.
Me: She seems good today, yeah?
Fred: Oh, yeah, she's good today.

Fred turned and walked from the kitchen to Mom's chair. Ashley, Andrew, and Mom were making small talk. I followed him to her chair and watched as he put a hand on her shoulder. She reached up and rubbed his hand and smiled.

Fred: You gonna show them?
MIL: Show them what?
Fred: (reaching inside her collar to reveal a new necklace) Your Christmas gift!
MIL: Oh, yeah...See? (holding up the charm on the necklace).

We all leaned in for a closer look. There was an exchange of ohhhs and ahhhs. Mom looked down at the charm and rubbed her thumb over it, then looked up to Fred.

MIL: Yep, he sure does like me, huh?
Me: (chuckling) He sure does, Ma. You got a good one there.
MIL: Uh huh.

There it was, she was back. Her eyes revealed a moment of the woman I had grown to love so much over the last twenty-nine years. I looked over my shoulder. Andrew had his arm around Ashley's waist as they watched Mom and Fred. I wondered if they saw her, too. I secretly thanked God for the gift of Mom, albeit only for a moment.

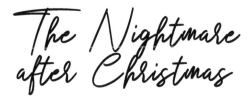

The Nightmare after Christmas

Connecticut

Boxing Day 2017

I yawned so wide my eyes watered, I shook my head and poured water into the coffeepot and yawned again. I heard the dogs at the back door. I waved at them to give me a second but then sighed heavily and put the pot down. I let them in. It was bitter cold, my coffee could wait a moment. I opened the door and the icy wind bit my face as I shooed the dogs in. I couldn't help but wonder what the temperature was in Naples that morning.

As I finished making the coffee, I mentally started to plan our day. Since our family trip to Naples had been abruptly canceled, we had decided on a lazy day. We planned to spend the day in our PJs watching corny Christmas movies. I was going to make a great roast dinner for us with all the "fixins" and we would just be with each other as a family, something that didn't happen often enough anymore.

Ashley crept into the family room as I was loading up the stove with wood.

Ashley: Mornin', Mama. Ohhh it's so toasty in here! (hugging herself tightly)
Me: Uh huh, it sure is. Hey, I was just thinking about dinner later, do you have a side dish you want to make?

145

Ashley: Yep, I have Brussels sprouts and potatoes I'm gonna roast.

Me: (turning my nose up a bit) Brussels sprouts?

Ashley: Yeah! (rubbing her belly) Yummy in my tummy. You'll like them, I promise.

Me: We'll see (rolling my eyes). I'm looking forward to a nothing day. How about you?

Ashley: Yeah, PJs all day!

Me: Sorry about Florida…

Ashley: It's okay, we'll get there another time. We just want to spend time with you and Daddy.

I pulled her in for a hug. This little treasure, now twenty-five years old, could still melt me into a bucket of mush. The back door opened and Joe stomped through.

Joe: Brrrrrr! It's cold out there!

Ashley: Hi Daddy!

Joe: Hey!

I watched his tired face light up like the Christmas tree I had just turned on. Joe is an amazing dad; our children are his world. A day of laziness would do him a world of good. I expected he would nod off on the sofa at some point, after all he was coming off a twenty-four-hour shift, but nevertheless it was going to be a great day.

Joe: Joey get off to work okay?

Me: Yeah, he left around 5:30. Said he'll be back around 12:30 or so. I told him we'd plan on the roast for late afternoon. I think he'll pick up Emily after he gets out of work.

Joe: That'd be good. I'm going to change.

Me: I'll get you coffee.

Joe reached down to give the dogs a round of Daddy lovin' before he headed upstairs. I heard the floorboard creak as Andrew stepped into the kitchen. He'd been feeling under the weather for most of Christmas day. Today his hair was a tousled mess, but he looked well rested and more himself.

Me: Hey there! How you feelin'?

Andrew: Wow, so much better. I should, I slept twelve hours straight!

Me: So glad to hear that. Can I get you anything?

Andrew: Nah...

Ashley: Want me to make you tea? It's a PJ day! (hopping on her toes like a five-year-old, giggling and laughing)

Me: Don't ever grow up, Baby.

Joe returned to the kitchen and I handed off his coffee. He looked relaxed and a little tired, but I didn't see stress in his face. Yesterday I had shared how great Mom was, and I was sure that had lifted a huge weight off his shoulders, at least temporarily.

Ashley: Good job, Daddy! I see you're sportin' your Christmas jammies!

Joe: Of course I am!

For the past twenty-five years, I had bought Christmas jammies for the kids and Joe. Each Christmas morning they all had new jammies on while they opened gifts. It was a silly little tradition, but during times like this when things were so unsettled, it was so good to have a little something we could all count on, even if it was only jammies.

We retired to the family room. Ashley curled up on one sofa with Andrew, while Joe and I settled into the other. The stove crackled as we sipped our coffees and just enjoyed being in the moment. Ashley started looking for corny Christmas movies while Joe and Andrew predicted the entire plot of every Hallmark Christmas movie ever made. The Christmas tree twinkled behind Ashley and Andrew while laughter filled the room. I thought, *God is good. Life is good.*

We were forty minutes into our movie when Joe's phone rang. Our eyes locked as he picked up the phone.

Joe: Hi Fred!...Okay, what's going on?

Joe put his coffee on the table and placed his other hand over his ear. I motioned to Ashley to turn down the volume as Joe walked out of the room.

Joe: Where is she now?…uh huh…how long?

I looked over to Ashley and Andrew and my heart sunk. My heart began to break. I knew our day was not going to happen, I could tell by the tone of Joe's voice as he left the room. Something had gone very wrong.

I knew the next steps far too well. I pulled myself off the sofa to go replace my festive PJ bottoms with pants. As I climbed the stairs, Joe passed me going down the staircase, still on the phone, his jammies also replaced with blue jeans. I hesitated on the fifth step.

Me: Let me at least put my pants on. Is she okay?
Joe: (ending his call) I don't know. Fred said she had explosive diarrhea over-
    night and now he can't get her up.
Me: Oh no. Okay, get me a fresh bottle of cleaner and a roll of paper towels.
    Oh, and a set of gloves. I'll be right down.
Joe: Okay.

I returned to the family room to find Joe giving Ashley and Andrew a report on what he knew. Ashley asked a few questions that he just couldn't answer yet.

Joe: We'll let you know as soon as we know something. Please keep the stove
    going; it's so cold out there.
Andrew: We got it (waving us out of the room). Go…go…GO!
Me: (exchanging a few quick hugs) I'm sorry. Maybe we'll be right back!
Ashley: It's okay, Mama. Go make sure everything's okay!

The ride was short, 3.4 miles to be exact, but it felt as if we were traveling clear across the country. I looked across the front seat of the truck and saw that the cloud of stress had returned to my love's face, but at least we were together. We were always best as a team. I didn't know what to do, so I filled the empty air with more questions. I quickly realized *that* was a bad idea. It didn't relieve his tension, it only added to it. We rounded the corner into Fred's driveway and the truck tires spun on the icy hill. Joe took a deep breath and rolled the truck back. He locked in the four-wheel-drive and made it easily up the hill. He was opening his door before the truck was even in park. I warned him to watch his step on the driveway, which was probably icy, yet somehow, he was almost to the door before I finished my warning. I grabbed the cleaning supplies out of the back seat and headed in myself.

I found Fred and Joe in the bedroom. The sheets had been stripped from the bed, Mom was lying on a bare mattress, naked, under the one blanket. Joe tried to assess her, although all he was getting from her was moaning and mumbling about hurting. He stood and turned to Fred.

Joe: Fred, how long ago did she get sick?
Fred: Well, she got up in the middle of the night and…had…ya know…(waving at his backside) all over the bathroom.
Joe: Mom (leaning down and shaking her gently). Mom?
Fred: She won't get up. She's been like this a little while.
Joe: (picking up her wrist and looking at his watch) How long?

I walked toward the bathroom with the gloves, paper towels, and cleaner, ready to take on whatever was there to meet me.

Fred: I cleaned it all up already.
Me: Sorry, Fred. I would have done that.
Joe: Ma, can you sit up for me?
MIL: (groaning) I…I…don't…I don't know.
Fred: I'm sure she's okay.…
Me: Did she throw up too?
Fred: No…just the backside.

Joe did a series of assessments. As I watched, I instinctively knew something was going very wrong. Joe guided me over to her as he covered her with the blanket again.

Joe: See if you can at least get a shirt on her. I've got to call the ambulance. Fred, she's gotta go in. There's too much going on.
Fred: I think she'll be fine.
Me: (clearing my throat) Uh…
Joe: (shooting a quick "I've got this" look in my direction) We can't take that chance…it's better just to have her checked out.
Fred: Well, I guess…

Joe and Fred left the bedroom. I stroked Mom's forehead for a moment. Her eyes were closed, she was laboring to breathe and winching in pain. I noticed her lips seemed slightly blue. I held her hand and noticed her fingertips were cold and slightly blue, too. I held her hand for a moment, thinking it may bring her some comfort.

Me: Mom? Joe would like you to get dressed. Can you help me with that?
MIL: Huh? (opening one eye).
Me: Can you sit up for me so I can put a nightshirt on you?
MIL: (beginning to sit, with my help) Ouch! (eyes popping wide open) Argh... that hurts! Oh, that hurts so bad.
Me: (gently laying her back) What hurts Mom? Can you point to what hurts?
MIL: Everything...everything hurts...but my back my back hurts most... ohhhhh...(panting) it hurts.

I stepped out into the main room. Joe was on the phone, requesting a medic from the dispatcher. He lifted his chin toward me and covered the phone.

Joe: Call Dave?
Me: Okay. I'm going to try again to get her shirt on, but she's now complaining of back pain.

He nodded in acknowledgment and continued talking with the dispatcher. I returned to the bedroom. I squatted next to the bed and gently brushed the hair from her eyes.

Me: Mom, I know you're not comfortable, and we're gonna figure out why you feel the way you do. Okay?
MIL: (groaning) Arghhhh...

I took a deep breath and stood up. I pulled at her dresser drawer, which scraped and squeaked as it opened. I looked over my shoulder and watched Mom, her face was knotted in pain. I moved aside the crumpled tissues and found a long night shirt. I shook it out and turned on my heel to look down at her. With a deep breath and a quick prayer for strength, I slid my arm under her large frame. I knew I couldn't possibly pick her up, but maybe by guiding her I could get her to sit up.

Me: Here we go, Ma (putting some pressure under her shoulder blades to help guide her up).

MIL: (groaning) Wwwwwhhhattt?!

Me: Help me out here, Ma. Can you sit up so I can get you dressed?

She opened one eye and leaned heavily against my hand as I pushed hard to help her sit upright. She was sweaty, her face was ashen, and she was laboring hard to breathe.

Me: (straining to lift her large frame) That's my beautiful girl.

Traditionally that got me a smile. That day, however, she didn't even open her eyes. Her focus was clearly just on breathing. I gently pulled open the neck of the night shirt and slid it over her head.

Me: Mom, can I have your arm? I want to slip it…

MIL: Arghhhh…oh that hurts…no, no, no…

Me: What hurts, Mom? Talk to me, your arm?

MIL: Yessss…

Me: Okay, I'll be gentle…

As she moaned and cried, I, as gingerly as possible, pulled her arms though the shirt. I laid her back against the pillows as she tried to catch her breath.

Me: Okay, one more thing, Mom. We need to get some underwear on you.

I unfolded the disposable underwear and positioned it so I could slide her legs in. I lifted up one leg and discovered she needed to be cleaned up a little more before we could continue. As I did so, I thought, *Thank God she won't remember this, she would be mortified.* She was able to briefly lift her backside up and I quickly slid on the underwear.

My first mission was accomplished, she was dressed. I recognized a sense of uneasiness in the room, more than the typical apprehension found when a medical emergency played out before you. This was different. I felt something shifting, something was happening, and I couldn't put my finger on what it was.

I could hear Joe's voice behind me rattling off stats to what I assumed was a dispatcher. I turned and looked at him. He was watching Mom intently. He covered the mouthpiece.

Joe: Go call Dave
Me: Okay.

I left the bedroom and stood in front of the large glass windows overlooking the driveway and called my brother-in-law Dave. I gave him what little information I had and asked him to reach out to Scot, too. I cut the conversation short, as I wanted to get back to Mom as quickly as I could. I knew she was scared.

As I disconnected our call, I watched the ambulance that had arrived in the driveway. Two EMTs were unloading the stretcher. Behind me I heard footsteps on the stairs. I looked over my shoulder to see one of our local EMTs, and friend, crest the top step.

Tom: Hey, Lisa (concern filling his face).
Me: Hey, Tom. She's down the hall, I'll show you the way.

I entered the bedroom and Joe was on the phone with Ashley, asking for verification on Mom's complete med list. He gave Tom a nod and a "One minute" gesture and left the room.

Me: Mom? (stroking her arm lightly) Hey, Beautiful.

Mom opened her eyes a bit.

Me: This is my good friend Tom. He's going to take a look at you and most likely take you for a ride to the hospital.
MIL: (weakly) Okay…
Me: I'll be right here (turning to see Joe re-enter). Oh, look, here's Joe too. We're here, Mom.

I stepped back as a paramedic and two more EMTs entered the room. I watched and answered questions that were directed to me. I watched Joe carefully as he assessed what the techs were reporting between themselves. He assisted where he could, without overstepping, and made a few comments. Joe is well respected in his field, this crew listened carefully to his commentary. It brought me great comfort knowing they were including him in their assessment.

I watched Fred, struggling to understand what I was reading on his face. Was it worry? Frustration? Fear?

The EMTs packed Mom into a chair to carry her down the fourteen stairs out to the waiting ambulance. She didn't understand why she was being tied down as the straps were tightened around her. Tom explained the straps were to keep her safe as Joe and I tried to reassure her. Her eyes got a little wild, so Joe stepped up to her.

Joe: Mom, it's okay (taking her hand in his and stroking her arm). You're only
    in this to get down the stairs (kissing her forehead).

The compassion and patience he showed was admirable. I didn't understand how he wasn't falling apart, how was he so calm? Then I realized, he had flipped that switch to paramedic mode because that was what was needed right then. I watched as he gently released her hand, the stairs creaked and popped as they lowered her down the stairwell. Joe turned to me and rattled off a list of instructions that fell on deaf ears momentarily. There was a strong sting rising in my eyes, I blinked hard to shake it back.

Joe: Honey? Hey! You hear me?
Me: (shaking my head in acknowledgment) Yeah, go, I'll meet you at the
    hospital.

He turned quickly and descended the stairs.

I looked around, trying to fully grasp what had just transpired. As I let my shoulder rest against the stairwell wall, I noticed the aftermath left by the emergency crew. A series of puddles of melted snow, peppered with sand and a few driveway stones were littered throughout the area. A used surgical glove, one of the EMTs must have dropped, lay on the floor. The quiet was deafening. I pushed myself off the wall and climbed the last two steps, swiped up the glove and pulled a healthy portion of paper towels off the dispenser. As my foot pushed the paper towels through the puddles, the back door slammed. I glanced down the stairs as I heard them groan with Fred's weight as he grasped the handrail to make the climb.

Fred: I'll do that.
Me: It'll only take me a minute. I won't be able to get in to see her for a bit. You know how those ERs are.
Fred: Yeah, well…she'll be fine.
Me: (swallowing hard) Yeah she will.
Fred: I'm going to the barn, we need more wood.

There seemed to be an air of dismissiveness in his tone.

Me: Okay, be careful. I'm going to head out, want me to call Vi to see if she can come clean?

Vi is Joe's brother Dave's wife, and I had mentioned a few times that she'd be willing to help, but Fred was having none of it.

Fred: No…no, I'm fine.

Fred looked down at the floor and shook his head. He lifted his chin while he skated his eyes sideways at me, letting out a soft, gruff sigh. As he turned his back, I tried to read his reaction.

Me: I'm going to head to the hospital, I'll call the kids and update them. Do you want me to call you when we know something? Maybe when you can visit?
Fred: (sharply) No, thank you.

My heart ached for Mom. Over the years she had been with Fred, she had a few hospital stays and he never visited. His reasoning was that hospitals "made him uncomfortable." I knew she would most likely not remember if he visited, but I suspected she would know something was missing. His not visiting felt selfish to me. I tried to remember Joe's philosophy that our capacity to handle Mom was different than others, that we couldn't judge. He always told me that we just needed to accept their comfort level.

Me: Okay, then (working hard to keep my tone light), I'm going to go.

Fred nodded, raised his hand, and dropped it abruptly as he rounded the corner.

Me: (quietly) Bye.

Red Sky in the Morning...

Connecticut

December 27, 2017

The alarm screamed, jolting me awake. My eyes burned and my head pounded from lack of sleep. I slid my arm across Joe's side of the bed, the sheets were cold and lacked the typical rumple he left after a night's sleep. Then I remembered, of course his side of the bed was crisp, he'd spent the night in the ER with Mom. It had been after midnight when Joe sent me home, there were still no answers, more tests to run, and no room for her. It had been an all-hands-on deck during the day. Joe's brothers Dave and Scot had spent a few hours sitting with Mom, giving us a little time to ourselves.

I rubbed my eyes with the back of my hand, knowing it was the worst thing to do for this aging skin. Although the temporary relief was worth it. I turned my face toward the window, taking in the changing skyline. The juxtaposition of pink and red jagged lines of the sunrise against the cobalt blue dawn sky was mesmerizing.

Red sky in the morning, sailors take warning…

I dragged myself from bed and threw on some clothes. I headed down to the kitchen, where the aroma of coffee greeted me.

Ashley: Morning, Mama (handing me a cup of steaming gold).

Me: Hey, Baby (yawning). You're up early.
Ashley:…Yeah, Andrew and I need to head home today.

I sipped the coffee as my eyes started to sting with tears. The logical, sensible mama in me knew I couldn't keep them here. The selfish, childlike side of me wanted to stomp my feet and throw a hissy fit.

Me: I figured as much.

A tear escaped. I wiped it away, quickly muttering "shit" under my breath.

Ashley: Oh, Mommy (her face filling with concern).
Me: I'm just tired, Baby. I'm upset we aren't in Florida right now, I'm frustrated we don't have answers about Grandma, and I'm worried about Daddy. He has to be exhausted…and I know we have some decisions to make.

She took my coffee cup from my hand and wrapped me in a hug. It was warm, it was strong, and it offered some short-lived comfort.

Ashley: Everything will be okay, Mama. Grandma has you and Daddy.
Me: (nodding my head) Yep, yep she does.

I studied the beautiful woman standing before me. My job was to be her rock. How did the tables turn?

Me: Baby, how about pancakes? I have frozen blueberries!?
Ashley: (rubbing her belly) Yummy in my tummy. I'll take my shower then wake Andrew up. He'll like that, too.
Me: I have chocolate chips too! Joey likes chocolate chips.
Ashley: Mom, Joey left for work at 5:30 this morning.
Me: Oh! I didn't make him lunch! I didn't even say goodbye to him…

The realization that I had slept late and basically forgot about my own son was too much. The flood gates opened. I turned quickly toward the sink; my shoulders pulled forward as a large, hard lump filled the back of my throat. I pinched the bridge of my nose and let the tears flow. Ashley laid a reassuring hand on my shoulder and pulled me into her arms again. She let her own tears escape, acknowledging our sadness, our losses. She pulled away and ripped two paper towels off the dispenser.

Ashley: Here, ugly cries need something sturdier than a tissue!

A smile crept across my face as I blew my nose and started to laugh. Ashley was right, it was an ugly cry, but it was a good cry all the same.

Me: (chuckling) Ugly cries are good for the soul sometimes (wiping my nose again). Go take your shower, Baby.
Ashley: You okay?
Me: Yeah, I am.

As I scooped the last pancake off the griddle, the back door opened and in walked Joe.

Me: Hey, how is she?
Joe: Sleeping, Scot came down to sit with her for a while.
Me: What did the doctors say?
Joe: UTI, but there's more going on…

I made my way around the counter and wrapped my arms around him. His coat was cold but his cheeks were warm. I held him tight, knowing that we are always stronger together.

Joe: (pulling back and waving his hand over the empty griddle) What's all this?
Me: Ashley and Andrew are heading home today.

He looked down at the floor.

Joe: I'm sorry.
Me: For what?!
Joe: This has been a crappy Christmas. The kids have given up so much.
Me: Stop, okay? (reaching to caress his arm) Just stop that. We raised good kids, they understand.
Joe: (shaking his head) I need a shower.

Joe's face was red, and he looked like he wanted to escape. He turned and exited the kitchen, leaving a sadness in the room. As I poured another cup of coffee, my phone chimed. I picked it up and another reality was staring back at me—my business.

It was a text from Katie asking if we could reschedule a meeting for the next day at 10:00 a.m.

I did a quick assessment in my head, *Ashley and Andrew are going home today, Joey will be working tomorrow, Joe's off tomorrow so if Mom needs something he'll be around.* I sent a return text to Katie confirming that it was fine and that I would be in later that day. She told me to take my time and she'd see me when I got there.

I returned the phone to the counter as Ashley and Andrew dropped their bags on the floor outside the kitchen. I felt another wave of emotions and told myself, *Pull it together!* I also realized much of what was happening to me emotionally was due to the intense past few months and lack of sleep.

We did our best to enjoy breakfast, to cherish the time we had together. It was short lived, Joe was feeling the pressure to return to the hospital and while the kids were nothing short of awesome, I was certain they, too, wanted to escape the uneasy, uncertain environment they had lived in for the past few days.

Joe: (sliding his chair back from the table) I've got to get back to the hospital.
Ashley: We're going to get going too.
Me: I need to get in the shower too. I have to stop by the studio. Honey, I'll come by the hospital in a little while and check on Mom. I'll call you on my way to see if you need coffee or a snack.

In a blink of an eye the house was silent. The wind rattled against the kitchen window as I placed the last dish in the dishwasher. Despite being in the warm house, a chill ran up my spine, and an uneasy feeling washed over me.

As promised, I made the visit to the hospital. Joe had finally secured Mom a room and she was settled in. His brother Scot had stayed for a few hours; Dave had checked in and had offered to sit with Mom after he finished at work. Fred, although we had reached out, didn't visit. His response was that he didn't like hospitals and that she'd be home soon and he'd see her then. I wondered if she missed him; she hadn't asked once for him. I looked over at Joe, he was leaning against the heater under her window.

Joe: I think she'll be fine tonight. She's in a room and Dave will be here.
Me: I can come back tonight for a while too.
Joe: No, let Dave sit with her. He wants to be here.
Me: Will he stay all night? You said she was restless last night. . .
Joe: I don't know, maybe she'll be better, you know, in her own room now...

Joe set his jaw and chewed on his bottom lip as he watched Mom sleeping. I could see the wheels turning in his head. We'd been dancing around the difficult conversation we knew we had to have. Could Mom even go back home? The fall earlier this month has made us start thinking differently. Joe had made an appointment with the social worker from the hospital the next day to discuss our options.

Joe: Maybe she'll be okay. Although it wouldn't be a bad idea to have him stay, if she wakes up she might be scared. I'll ask him.
Me: I can stay if he can't.
Joe: No, you have a presentation tomorrow.
Me: Let's see how the evening shakes out. How about you head home now, take a nap before you have to get ready for work. I'll wait for Dave.
Joe: I'll go soon.
Me: Honey? (crossing the room and placing my hand on his arm) You need to get some rest, you aren't going to be any good for the guys without a little sleep.

Joe gave me a dismissive shrug, although I knew he knew I spoke the truth. He pushed off the heater with a quick shove.

Joe: You're right, plus I think I'm going to need to get FMLA paperwork in place.
Me: Go on (kissing his cheek), I'll wait for Dave. He'll be here in a few hours.

Joe leaned over Mom and kissed her. He paused and stroked her hair back as she slept. I watched him exit the room and I settled into the chair with my laptop.

MIL: Hmmmm? Hey?
Me: (rising from the chair and approaching the side of her bed) Hey, Beautiful, how you doin'?
MIL: (squinting at me) Okay…

Mom closed her eyes as she gently began to snore. I returned to my computer and worked for a few hours as Judge Judy kept me company before the local news began and Dave walked in.

Dave: Hi (just above a whisper). How is she?
Me: Hey there, she's slept almost the entire time I've been here.
Dave: How long have you been here?
Me: I came by around 1:30 or so, I sent Joe home to take a nap before work, he left at 2:00…I think.
Dave: Well, I can stay for a bit.
Me: I'm not sure she should be alone tonight.
Dave: I'll stay.
Me: The night?

Avoiding an affirmative answer, Dave asked about the kids and how our Christmas was. I shared that Joe worked a twenty-four-hour shift on Christmas Day, so it wasn't much of a holiday, but the kids and I made the best of it. I chose not to rehash the loss of our lazy day in our jammies or the fact that there was no family dinner and no family trip to Florida.

Me: Ya know what? I'm going to head out if you're all set? If I leave now, there's a slim chance I can see Joe before he leaves. I want to make sure he has dinner.
Dave: Sure, yeah, of course.

I reached up to hug his tall, lanky frame. I wanted him to know I loved him.

Me: I'll call you later to check on her.
Dave: Okay.

I slid behind the wheel of the car; the leather seats were so cold it penetrated through my winter coat. The clock on the dash confirmed my fear that I would not make it home before Joe left for work. I love Joe's brothers, but sadly Mom's illness had created some tension between us. I had yet to understand why, but it was there. A tear escaped, I quickly wiped it away. The car roared to life, and I started the escape to home, albeit temporary.

The evening moved along quickly. Joey decided to spend the evening at Emily's, so I had the house to myself. I curled up on the sofa and lost myself in the *Outlander* series. Claire and Jamie's love story was a good distraction. On television, a gruesome battle scene ended. As the television screen showed the the sun rising over the carnage on the battlefield, the skyline was a blaring red.

Red sky in the morning, sailors take warning.

I reflected on that morning's sunrise, which admittedly felt like three days ago, as our old Regulator clock chimed 9:00 p.m.

I texted Dave to see how Mom was doing.

Text from Dave: She's sleeping. I think I'm going to head home.
Text from Me: I don't think she should be alone, she'll be scared if she wakes up.
Text from Dave: I have to work tomorrow.

I stared at the phone and thought, *Yep, so do I.*

Text from Me: Can you wait till I get there? I'll leave right now.
Text from Dave: K.

I sent both Joey and Joe texts that I am heading to the hospital. Joe responded that he thought if Dave couldn't stay, that she'd be fine. My gut was telling me I needed to be there. I could remember nights when Mom had stayed with us after other hospital stays and she would wake up not knowing where she was.

She became disoriented and frightened. She just had a fall less than a month ago, I knew I needed to go.

As I entered Mom's room, Dave was sitting in the chair next to her bed. His eyes were bloodshot, I could see he was tired.

Me: (whispering) Hey, thanks for waiting.
Dave: She's pretty much slept the entire time. She woke up to eat, then went back to sleep.
Me: Maybe she'll sleep all night.
Dave: She probably will. Sorry I can't stay. I'm exhausted and have to work in the morning.
Me: It's okay, I got this. I have a presentation in the morning, and Joe is meeting with the social worker. Is Vi still on school vacation? Can she come sit with Mom in the morning?
Dave: I'll check with her (rising out of the chair).
Me: Please, let me know if she can be here by seven. That will give me time to get home, shower, and regroup for my meeting.
Dave: I'll check with her; I don't know what she has planned.

A quick smile crossed my lips, as I selfishly thought, *Seriously? Can you guys make some sacrifices too?* I shook it off. I remembered Joe telling me everyone has their own tolerance levels. We needed to understand that this journey was affecting different family members in different ways, we could not judge, we could not be angry...we just had to accept whatever help they could offer.

Me: Well...let me know (reaching up for a hug).
Dave: I will...and thank you. I think she'll be fine tonight, but I feel better with you here.

Dave took a few steps to the side of the bed. I stepped back, giving him a few minutes of privacy with his mom. He brought his face close to hers, his right hand gently stroked her hair while his left held her hand. A soft smile graced her lips. Dave whispered against her cheek, and the smile grew. I heard a throaty chuckle rise in his throat. As he rose above her, she puckered her lips into a kiss, Dave dropped his cheek to accept it.

He turned to me and pulled me in for another hug.

Dave: Thanks again (rubbing my back). You're the best.
Me: Of course.
Dave: I told Mom to watch out for Nurse Ratchet tonight (chuckling). She even smiled. Yeah, okay I've gotta go. I've got to be at work by 6:30.
Me: Go, just let me know what Vi can do.

As Dave closed the door, I settled into the stiff hospital recliner and used the remote to flip through channels. Sleep found me quickly, despite the uncomfortable chair. I was awakened with a start when I heard Mom arguing with a nurse.

MIL: Stop that…do *not* touch me!
Nurse: Ms. Zieroth, please…I need to take your vitals.
MIL: I said LEAVE. ME. ALONE!

I jumped from the chair and scurried to Mom's side. I raised my hand as a signal to the nurse to give me a moment.

Me: Hey, Mom! (caressing her arm) It's okay. I'm here with you.
MIL: (eyes wide and wild) What the HELL do you want?

My head snapped back. I exchanged a concerned look with the nurse across the bed. Behind me the local weatherman reported rising temps, strong winds, and rain throughout the evening.

Me: Mom? Hey, look at me, Beautiful (stroking her hand).
Nurse: Ms. Zier…(picking up her wrist).
MIL: (snapping her hand away) Don't…I said…No…NO!
Me: (looking at the nurse) How about I work on calming her down and you come back in a little while?
Nurse: I have to take her vitals.
Me: (looking to avoid an argument) I get it, can you come back in a little bit? Clearly she's upset.
MIL: Don't…I don't want it!
Me: Yes, Mom, I know.

Nurse: She can't be yelling either. Other patients are trying to sleep (hastily grabbing the blood pressure cuff off the side of the bed).

I sternly looked at the nurse. Under my breath I muttered, "No shit, Sherlock."

Nurse: I'm sorry, what did you say?
MIL: No SHIT! You heard her...No SHHHIIITTTT!
Me: Okay, Mom...sssshhhh, we've got to keep our voices down.

The nurse turned on her heel and left. Nurse Ratchet. Of course we would get her tonight!

Me: Mom?
MIL: What do YOU want?!
Me: I'm here to keep you company. You know, you and me...we're two peas in a pod.
MIL: Where am I? WHY am I here? You.... YOU can't...can't make...HERE?
Me: Shhh, remember other patients are sleeping.

I grabbed my phone and texted Joe.

Text from Me: I'm at the hospital with Mom.
Text from Joe: ?? I thought Dave was there.
Text from Me: Did you miss my text?

MIL: Do YOU hear me? What is this? (picking at the tape on her IV).
Me: Mom don't do that (pulling her hand away).

Text from Me: He had to go home...too tired...has to work in a.m.
Text from Joe: She should be okay, go home.
Text from Me; Yeah, not so much. We're off to a rough start...can I request a sedative?

MIL: Where's Frrr...Where's Fred ?...

Me: Home, Mom. You need to rest (watching my phone).
Text from Joe: You can try...call coming in.

I looked to the ceiling, then dropped my head in frustration. Sometimes I hated his job. I needed him to answer *my* questions. I'd grown to understand being second fiddle to the job, but that night I wanted to be first string.

MIL: Hey…HEY…
Me: Yes, Mom?

She dropped her head against the pillow and closed her eyes. I studied her for a moment. Was she going back to sleep? I wished I had a better understanding of what was going on in that head of hers.

I slowly backed away from the bed and momentarily reminisced of taking the same steps putting my babies to sleep at night. I made my way to the recliner, which creaked as I started to sit down. I hesitated and braced myself mid-sit, hoping to not wake her. She didn't stir, so I released my body and sunk into the chair. In my own uneasiness, I rested my head against the headrest and closed my eyes.

I heard the squelch of the Velcro release on the blood pressure cuff and jolted awake. I watched as Nurse Ratchet stuffed the cuff into a rollaway stand. She glared at me over her reading glasses.

Nurse Ratchet: I see you calmed her down.
Me: (whispering) Yes…maybe she'll sleep…
Nurse Ratchet: (speaking in anything but a quiet bedside manner) Well, we
    have a full house tonight. I have a schedule to keep.

I nodded and watched Mom. I willed her to be good tonight, to behave, and sleep all night.

Nurse Ratchet: She seems to be out cold. I'll be back in a few hours. You're
    going to need to turn that down (nodding at the television), other patients
    are sleeping.

Behind me, Jimmy Fallon was barely audible on the television screen. I reached for the remote and turned Jimmy off completely.

Nurse Ratchet: Much better.

As she turned on her heel, the wheel on her rolling desk squealed and spun quickly.

MIL: Huh? What's...wha...Who's that?!
Me: (stroking her arm) Shhh. It's okay, Mom, I'm here.

She closed her eyes and drifted off to sleep again. I breathed a sigh of relief and returned to the chair. I looked at the ceiling and started my own little conversation with God. I thanked him for Nurse Ratchet, dripping with sarcasm, then asked Him for a quiet night. My prayers continued, I listed my gratitudes, asked Him to keep Joe safe tonight, and drifted off into a restless sleep.

MIL: Hey, BITCH!...You!...HEY!

The adrenaline surged alive in my veins as I grabbed the arms of the chair and jumped to a standing position. Mom was sitting straight up in bed, her eyes are wide, wild, and ablaze. The shadows cast over her face from the dim nightlight over her bed made her look frightening to say the least. I slowly made my way to the side of her bed, reaching across the bed rail to gently touch her arm.

Me: (speaking just above a whisper) Mom, it's okay...I'm here, what do you
    need?
MIL: I...I know you...YOU! (slapping my hand, hard) BITCH!

I pulled my hand back as if I touched a hot burner. The sting from her slap cut equally as deep.

Me: Ouch...Mom! Stop that!
MIL: Get outta here!
Me: (working hard to gather some composure) Shh...Mom, we have to be
    quiet! Other people are sleeping. It's okay (cautiously reaching across the
    rail again to her arm).
MIL: (snapping her arm away from my touch) I...I...(leaning forward toward
    me, glaring) I...geeeeettt you! I know what YOU do. I will NOT stand
    for YOU and your pretty pants coming here!

Me: Shhhh, Mom...the nurse is going to come.
MIL: I don't care!...I gotta go home...I need to...

Mom grabbed the rails of the bed and started shaking them. The racket radiated down the hall, summoning Nurse Ratchet.

Me: Shit, Ma...Come on! Please, shhhhhh!
MIL: Fuck you, BITCH!

The word *bitch* flew from her mouth, laced with hate and detest. Then she actually spit at me. As I wiped my face, Nurse Ratchet pushed the door open.

Nurse Ratchet: Keep your voices down!
Me: I'm sorry. Clearly she is having a hard time. Can we get a sedative, something to help her sleep and calm her down?
MIL: Don't you touch me.
Me: I think we need someth...
Nurse Ratchet: I'll call the doctor, but you need to do something.
Me: I'm doing the...
MIL: Get out of here...no...I'm going home (pushing Nurse Ratchet's arm off the rail).
Me: (looking at the nurse) How about you give that doc a call?

Nurse Ratchet nodded and left. Part of me wanted to follow her out, then head down to my car and home into my safe, warm bed.

Me: Okay, Mom. We're going to get you home soon, sound good?
MIL: (glaring at me) Grumph.

I knew I was telling her a big, fat lie, but I was hopeful that in ten minutes she wouldn't remember what I said. She settled into her pillow and closed her eyes. I looked at the clock, 2:28 a.m. I watched as the second hand clicked along. I counted off the hours until 7:00 a.m., four and half hours. Could I do this? I turned my attention back to Mom, who was now sleeping again. I hung my head, looking for my own escape as I stumbled back into the chair. Sleep didn't rescue me. I sat and watched the second hand click its way around the face of the clock.

Nurse Ratchet pushed the door open. I glanced at the clock, 3;12 a.m.

Nurse Ratchet: (speaking, finally, just above a whisper) The doctor just called in a sedative, I've ordered it from the pharmacy.

I mouthed the words *thank you* and offered up a set of praying hands. My experience with hospital pharmacies was not extensive, although I did know it would be at least an hour before we would get a delivery. The door creaked a bit as Nurse Ratchet left.

MIL: Huh? (her eyes partially opening)

I held my breath and watched her. She closed her eyes again and turned her head away, a soft snore escaped her lips. I listened to the repetitive click of the second hand on the clock and waited.

My eyes couldn't fight the sleep, they closed as my head fell forward only to snap back again. I struggled to focus on the clock, 3:53. a.m. A storm had whipped up outside. Wind and rain slammed against the window, seemingly mimicking the battle I was waging in that little hospital room. Through my fog of exhaustion, I heard Mom's bed rustling, it took me a moment to register where I was and what the sound was. I opened my eyes and focused on the bed. Mom was sitting up, picking the tape on her arm. I watched her for a moment before I realized it was the IV tape she was pulling at. I bolted out of the chair.

Me: (grabbing her arm) Mom, no! Don't pick at the IV!
MIL: (pulling her hand away) Don't touch me!
Me: I'm sorry, Mom, but you can't…

I never saw it coming. Her right hand swung across the bed and made contact with my cheek, it stung and burned. I stood, stunned.

MIL: That'll teach ya…bitch.
Me: (rubbing my face) That was uncalled for.
MIL: (snickering) No…

I searched for the woman I loved, I only saw a bitter, angry woman who thought I was someone else. We started a standoff, she watched me, I watched her. When she thought I wasn't paying attention, she'd pull at her IV and I'd start the battle again. Although now I was smarter and dodged any outbursts.

I glanced up at the clock, careful not to take my eyes away from Mom, 4:20 a.m. I reached across the bed for the call button and pressed it. The intercom jumped alive and so did Mom.

Woman on the intercom: Yes?
Me: Hello? Yes, can you check on Rosemary's sedative?
Woman on the intercom: Hold on, please.
MIL: Who the hell is THAT?
Me: The nurses' station.
MIL: What the hell do they want?
Me: (sarcastically) A night off from us...
MIL: What?
Me: Nothing, Mom.
MIL: I don't know what you're doing here.
Me: Me neither...

The door opened and Nurse Ratchet rolled in her rolling torture table, at least that was what it appeared to be that night.

Nurse Ratchet: Rosemary, I need to take your vitals again.

All I could think was, *Are you kidding me?*

MIL: Don't touch me! (pulling away and looking up at me) Make her leave.
Me: So now I'm your friend?
MIL: What the hell are you talking...OUCH!

Mom reacted as the nurse lifted her hand to place the blood pressure cuff.

Me: It's okay, Mom, she's not hurting you.
MIL: YES. she. IS!
Me: (looking at the nurse) Any word on that sedative?

Nurse Ratchet: They are busy tonight; it will be here soon.

By some grace of God, we made it through the blood pressure and other tasks. Nurse Ratchet left and Mom fell into her pillow again, staring at the ceiling. I watched her carefully, wondering if we were in the clear. As the thought passed through my head, the battle began again, "Mom don't touch..." and it's a swing and a miss. At 5:10 a.m. Nurse Ratchet returned with a syringe. I looked to the heavens with a prayer of thanks.

Nurse Ratchet: This should help (pushing the needle into the IV).
MIL: What are you doing?
Me: Helping the Sand Man arrive, Ma (rubbing my eyes).
Nurse Ratchet: She shouldn't be on this floor.

The nurse dropped the syringe into the box above Mom's bed and leaves.

MIL: Yea, I should...(groggily) I shouldn't...

Mom rested her head on her pillow as sweet slumber enveloped her. I looked at the clock, 5:16 a.m. I turned and collapsed into the chair. I picked up my phone and set the alarm for 6 a.m. I noticed three text messages from Joe.

Text 12:45 a.m.: Hey sorry, try to get a sedative if she's not sleeping.
Text 1:09 a.m.: Did you get the sedative?
Text 2:57 a.m.: Just got back from a call, you must have gotten the sedative, I'll call you in the morning.

The alarm chirped at 6 a.m. A warm yellow line screamed across the horizon, announcing the rising sun. I hit "end" on my phone and checked my text messages.

Text from Dave: Vi can be there by 7:30, maybe sooner.

I scrolled through emails. Katie confirmed the presentation for that morning, another email notified me of a backorder on fabric, and one about price increases scheduled for January 1. Mom snored loudly as I watched her. I prayed she would never remember that night. I knew it would break her heart.

I turned on the morning news as Nurse Ratchet's replacement entered the room.

Nurse: (whispering) Good Morning, how is she doing?
Me: Sleeping finally.
Nurse: I heard it was a rough night. How are you doing?
Me: Tired (yawning), but glad to see the sun still came up this morning.
Nurse: It was a nice sunrise this morning, the sky was golden yellow, nice to see after last night's storm.

She gently cared for Mom, taking vitals, talking about the storm quietly. Mom doesn't even stir.

Nurse: Looks like the doctor's cocktail did the trick.
Me: The sleep will do her good.
Nurse: She'll be okay, why don't you go home, she'll sleep for hours.
Me: My sister-in-law is coming soon. I'll stay until she gets here.
Nurse: Can I get you anything? Coffee? Sue, our floor manager, makes a mean pot?
Me: Oh, that would be great.

My new angel left and quickly returned with a steaming cup of coffee, complete with milk on the side. If I had told her how I take my coffee, it didn't register. I watched the sun break over the buildings outside Mom's window. No red sky warnings that morning. I wondered if maybe we had turned the corner. As I drained the last drop of coffee, the door swung open.

Vi: Good Morning!
Me: Hey…

I crossed the room and welcomed Vi's warm hug. I held on probably a moment longer than I should. I just needed a little bit of love at that moment, so I selfishly took it in.

Vi: How is she?
Me: Rough night…but we got a sedative in her, so she should sleep for a few hours.

Vi: Oh, well I brought some magazines. I can stay 'til about 11, then I have some things to do.

Take it, Lisa. Take it with a smile.

Me: That's a huge help. Joe's getting off work soon; I'm sure he'll go home, take a shower, and head down.
Vi: Tell him not to rush.
Me: I know he has to meet with the social worker this morning, so I'm sure he'll be here by 9:30.

I crossed the room to Mom's bedside. Her mouth was wide open and deep sleep her salvation. I leaned down and kissed her forehead.

Me: (whispering) We made it through the night, Beautiful. I love you, sleep well. I'll see you later.

I exchanged a few additional pleasantries with Vi and left Mom's room. I walked out of the most difficult night of my life. I closed the door, leaned my head against the wall, and cried.

Nurse Angel was passing by and stopped to rub my shoulder gently. She whispered something about strength and love. I couldn't process what she was saying. My heart was breaking. I squared up my shoulders, smiled through the tears, and thanked her for her kindness.

As the hospital doors opened, the warm sun hit my face. I think about how it's time to put on my next hat, designer and business owner. I symbolically hang my caretaker hat, temporarily.

Captain and First Mate

Connecticut & Florida

January 2018

I stroked his hand with my thumb as he checked the rearview mirror on our way to the airport. Fatigue masked Joe's face, and guilt filled my heart. For the past week, Joe and I had been navigating uncharted waters. He was the captain, I his first mate. We'd been blessed with a stellar crew of deck officers dressed as social workers, a few experienced friends, and an amazing nursing staff. They had been encouraging and resourceful, despite some treacherous seas. Still, there, laid out before us, was an open sea, filled fifty-foot swells and scary sea monsters. I watched the cars pass on the highway as I played out events of the last month in my head: the fall, the accusations, this last hospital stay, and now the rehab center.

Me: What time are you meeting with Regency House?
Joe: 10:00 a.m., they have a team to review Mom's file.
Me: I land at 11:30, I'll call you to see how it went. Have you talked to Fred?
Joe: No.
Me: This is the right move.
Joe: I know.

We knew she couldn't go back to Fred's. We knew we couldn't take her to our house. Mom needed constant care, she needed someone to watch over her 24/7. I wished I could share that week's meetings with Joe, but I had lost too much time over the past four weeks and it was beginning to take its toll. Joe pulled the car to the curb at departures.

Joe: See you Saturday (leaning across for a kiss).
Me: I miss you already…love you.
Joe: Me too…love you, too.

The day passed quickly, I jumped into meetings and calls, working well past 7:30 p.m. before I called Joe.

Me: Hey, how did it go?
Joe: Okay.
Me: You seemed to be making good progress today.
Joe: Jen's been great, I just…

Jen was Joey's girlfriend Emily's mom, and she had been a huge help in advising us.

Me: Honey?
Joe: Maybe we can keep her at our house?

I hung my head, glad he couldn't see me. We'd been around and around on this. We'd even cleared out the living room, prepping, only to realize we really couldn't care for her properly, Not with us both working full time. I thought after the conversations with Jen and the social workers we had made our decision.

Me: We talked about this…
Joe: (cutting me off) I know we did! But how do I just leave my mother?
Me: Woah…easy. I know this is hard, but…
Joe: But what?! She's my mom…
Me: Okay, I know you're upset…
Joe: My brothers don't feel like this is necessary.
Me: (sighing) Well, they are her children, although I have a hard time saying they can have an opin…
Joe: (sharply) They have a right to an opinion.

I was a little taken aback by his reaction. The night before, as we discussed a permanent stay at Regency House, he had told me I should be an active participant in the decision-making process. I was confused and, selfishly, hurt.

Me: (quietly) You're right, they *do* have the right to have a say. Yet they aren't willing to step up and take her in.
Joe: Just stop, okay? She's their mother, too.

Silence filled the phone line. I was confused and not sure what to say or do. I wasn't there with him, he was left to do this on his own.

Me: When do we need to make a final decision? She has a few more weeks of rehab right?
Joe: I think so.
Me: I'll be home in a few days, why don't we have your brothers over and discuss it.
Joe: Maybe…

I changed the subject, looking for anything to lighten the mood building on that call. I had little success. We exchanged our I love yous and disconnected. I dropped the phone on the coffee table and leaned back into the sofa. I closed my eyes, wondering how we would manage if the decision was to move Mom home with us.

I leaned forward and picked up my phone and texted Joe.

Me: I love you…whatever you decide I'll support.
Joe: Whatever WE decide. I love you, too. Sorry I snapped.
Me: It's okay, we will make the best choice for Mom.

We Ping-Ponged back and forth over the week I was away, but upon my return we settled in on the decision that Regency House would become Mom's new home. A home we would find to be the ultimate fit for her, and for us.

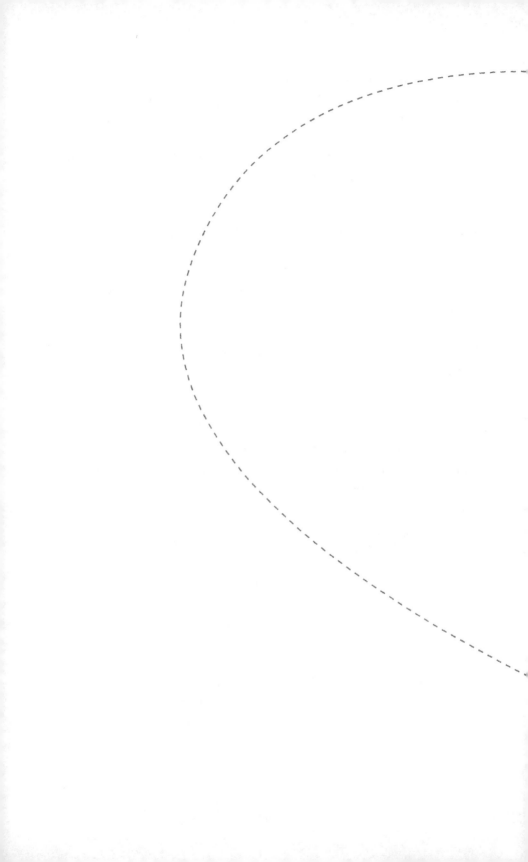

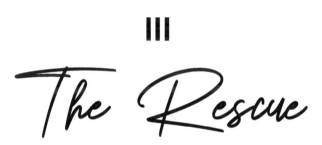

III

The Rescue

Help, Aid, and Support

Regency House

Connecticut

March 2018

I watched Mom sleep, she looked so peaceful. She was settling into this new home at Regency House. Megan, a nurse supervisor who had helped us immensely in getting Mom into Regency House guided us through the process and advocated fiercely for Mom. She also counseled Joe and me well when we needed her most. When Megan affectionately began to refer to Mom as "RoRo," we knew she was home.

While we were confident in our decision, it was not without cost. Fred never agreed to the path we ultimately took with Mom. He wanted to keep caring for her, but we felt she needed more care and that it would be too much for Fred (and us) to continue caring for her at home. Joe, as a paramedic, had years of exposure to facilities and felt strongly that Regency House was the right choice for his mom. Their Star Unit, a memory-care unit, would prove to be the perfect fit for her and us. We will always be thankful to Fred for the happiness he brought into Mom's life when they were together.

While things were better and I knew Mom was receiving the care she needed, I had admittedly been struggling over the past few months, leaving for weeks at a time was weighing on my heart. Joe had stood by my side, supporting me unconditionally as I built my design business. Juggling had always been something at which I thought I was pretty successful. Motherhood, wife, career, family, and friendships were in constant rotation, with me trying to catch each one at just the right moment and then toss it back into the loop. I chuckled to myself, replaying that image in my head, and seeing the kids as children, Joe in paramedic school, family celebrations, weddings, first birthdays, and even the difficult heartbreaking moments of illness and death as balls to keep in the air. I saw myself then gracefully moving the balls, even balancing on one foot occasionally to knock one into the rhythm. However, recently, that career ball was consistently occupying one hand, while the other kept moving every other ball. The balance was off, my travel was laced with guilt and heartache. I have always believed that in this juggling act of life there are glass balls and one rubber ball that would bounce if I dropped it. My career was that rubber ball. Mom also lived that juggling act, hers was laced with divorce, family dysfunction, and health challenges. She had said she didn't do it well, yet when I looked at the man she raised, I strongly disagreed.

I slid back into the chair, letting my head rest on the back. My feet were propped on the bed rail, I studied her face and let my mind wander. Mom and I had come a long way. I smiled as I remembered when Joe and I moved in with her six months after we were married. It was 1991 and we were struggling to make ends meet. Reluctantly, I accepted Mom's offer to live with her. I was worried about how I could share a household with her, yet grateful and bound and determined to make the best of the situation.

The memories flowed back of that first Sunday morning together…

I filled the coffeepot, looking out into the backyard. Joe was already up and mowing the lawn. I sighed deeply and looked at a pile of boxes by the dining room table that I needed to unpack or at least move into one of our rooms today. It had been almost a week since Joe and I had moved in with my mother in-law. Admittedly, I was feeling like a failure. Married less than six months and we couldn't make it financially on our own. I tried to remind myself that our country was experiencing a deep recession, that our timing to get married was just ill-planned. Yet I repeatedly heard in the back of my head all those naysayers that

said we were too young to get married, it would be a mistake, or we wouldn't make it. Now, a week into my second new home in six months, I was wondering if maybe I should have heeded the advice.

I heard the bathroom door close down the hall and thought, <u>Oh, she's up.</u> I quickly busied myself in the kitchen, wiping down counters, sweeping the floor, trying hard to show I was earning my keep.

I heard Mom shuffling down the hall in a morning stupor. I quickly pulled two coffee cups out of the cabinet and willed the pot to finish brewing.

Me: Morning!

I grabbed the coffeepot, partially brewed, and poured two cups of coffee. As I poured milk into my cup, I hesitated. <u>How does she take her coffee?</u> As I opened my mouth to ask, I heard the scraping and jingle of keys slide across the front table and the front door slam. I stood in the kitchen with two steaming coffee cups in hand, a little stumped. Who doesn't acknowledge a cheerful "Morning" greeting?

I cautiously leaned under the upper cabinet that separated the dining space and kitchen, craning my neck to look through the dining window. I saw Mom yawning and opening the car door. I wondered where she could be going on a Sunday morning. I knew she didn't go to church, she hadn't even had a cup of coffee yet. I quickly decided it wasn't really my business and poured the second coffee cup back into the pot.

I looked at the pile of boxes, what do I unpack? I mean, I don't need dishes, pots, or pans…although I couldn't find a salad bowl two days ago. I decided I'd take an inventory of what was in the kitchen and add our own to whatever was missing. One box was completely inventoried and unpacked and repacked when the front door opened with a bang, startling me a bit.

Me: *(leaning around the corner to see her) Oh, Gosh! Mom, you startled me!*
MIL: *Grumph.*

I watched as she dropped her keys on the table and her purse on the chair. I thought, Is she even going to say good morning? I was raised in a home where mornings were cheerful and happy. Over these first few months of marriage, Joe reminded me almost daily that Davenports are not morning people, which is fine,…but did that mean you can't acknowledge a "Good Morning"?

Me: *Hey there! Good morning!*

Nervously I started to babble…

Me: *I made coffee, can I pour you a cup? Here, I'll clear the table, so you can have a cup, maybe I can join you? Would you like that? If not that's okay too, coffee?*

She looked at me like my head was going to spin clear off my neck.

MIL: *Ummmm, I guess so.*
Me: *Great, hang on, I'll get you a cup. How do you take your coffee? Milk? I think I saw cream in the fridge. Do you need sugar? Or black? Or do you want me to pour the coffee and just have you fix it yourself? Some people are picky about their coffee? You picky about your coffee?*

She closed her eyes for a minute and shook her head. She opened her eyes and just stared at me.

Me: *Mom?*

MIL: Holy crap, how much coffee have you had?!

Me: Half a cup, there's plenty, I was just going to see if Joe wanted a cup too. I can see if he wants to join us. It looks like the back lawn is almost done. It would be nice. We can all sit together and have coffee. Yeah, I think that would be nice, don't you? Coffee together on a Sunday...

MIL: (holding up one hand) Whoa.

Me: What?

MIL: (waving me out of the way) I'll get my coffee.

Me: Okay, I'll freshen mine up too. Then we can sit...

MIL: Nope, I'll just have my coffee and sit with my paper.

Mom pulled the New York Times *out of a plastic shopping bag and dropped it on the counter. Dejected, I stepped aside, looking at the floor as she poured her coffee and yawned. She stepped past me with her coffee, scooped up the newspaper, and made her way into the family room. I listened as she sighed deeply and flopped into her recliner. I crept around the corner and watched her open the newspaper and take a sip of her coffee.*

Me: Mom?

MIL: Hmmmm? (not taking her eyes off her newspaper).

Me: Mom? I can make eggs and toast? Or maybe pancakes? Would you like pancakes? I can't jazz them up with anything. Yeah I can make pancakes or just eggs if you want. Just let me know.

MIL: (still looking at the paper) Tell you what, how about this. You leave me alone and let me read my paper and drink my coffee and you do what you want to do? Okay? Geeezzzeeee.

The heat rose quickly in my cheeks as I spun quickly to escape.

Me: (softly) Okay...

MIL: (almost too enthusiastically) Great!

I walked out the back door and stood on the deck, looking out at Joe making the last sweep with the lawn mower. As the steam

185

from my coffee cup filled my face, I thought, She hates me. *Why wouldn't she? I've invaded her home, when Joe and I married he was the last one to leave the nest. This gave Mom her own space for the first time in her life. Now here I was, turning her peaceful new life on its head.*

Joe climbed the deck stairs, wiping his forehead with his sleeve.

Joe: Hey.
Me: She hates me.
Joe: (confused) Huh? Who?
Me: Your mother. She hates me.
Joe: Hardly, she loves you!
Me: Oh yea? (scoffing) You should have seen her in there, she didn't even say good morning. I even offered to make her coffee for her. I offered eggs and toast or to make pancakes, I said they wouldn't be fancy, but they'd be good, or I could just make eggs and she (my lip quivering a bit) and she said (a tear escaping down my cheek) to just leave her ALONE!
Joe: (chuckling) I bet she did!
Me: What?!
Joe: We're not morning people, Honey. I've told you that. You are a little much to handle first thing in the morning.
Me: (wiping my tears) Well, she didn't have to be rude. I mean seriously, I was just trying to be nice. I know it's a lot having us here. I just wanted to make her coffee or some breakfast. I was just trying to be NICE!
Joe: (shaking his head dismissively) Oh, Honey.
Me: What?! (tears now flowing fast)
Joe: Relax, by noon she'll be fine.

He gently kissed my cheek and wiped a tear with his soft yet calloused thumb.

Joe: (resting his hand on my cheek) How about you get me a cup of coffee?

I reluctantly agreed, I didn't even want to go back into the house. Of course any twenty-three-year-old kid would have been a little gun shy. I opened the back door and quietly made my way around the kitchen pulling a mug out of the cabinet and pouring Joe's coffee. I picked up the fresh mug and peeked around the corner to see if Mom had softened. She was sitting in her chair, the newspaper folded into quarters, and her glasses hanging from the corner of her mouth as she held the paper close to her face. Her brow was furrowed in concentration, even I knew better than to interrupt her. I turned and tried to exit the kitchen quietly out the back door while holding two cups of hot coffee. I was not successful, the screen door slipped from my awkward grasp and slammed. I cringed as I heard Mom shriek.

I crossed the deck to where Joe was sitting on a ratty old lawn chair gazing over the railing and surveying the freshly cut grass.

Me: Crap.
Joe: What?
Me: Did you hear your Mom?
Joe: No.
Me: (handing Joe the cup of steaming coffee) I let the screen door slam; I think she came out of her skin.
Joe: Well, when she's doing that puzzle she's in another world.
Me: (taking a sip of my coffee) What puzzle?
Joe: The New York Times *crossword puzzle. She does it every Sunday. She can spend a good part of the day working on it.*
Me: (my eyebrows rising, impressed and in awe) Really? Does she finish it each week?
Joe: Pretty much. Sometimes I find it on the table with a few empty spaces, later in the week. She'll pick it up and stare at it for a bit, then put it back (taking a sip of his coffee and shaking his head). Then she'll get up from the family room, walk to the

table, pick up the paper, and fill in a blank space, she smiles like she's won lotto or something.

I sat back in my chair, sipping my coffee and looking out over the backyard of the house where Joe was raised. I thought about the woman I barely knew in the family room, how she opened her home to Joe and I when we needed it most. I needed to remember I was in her house, and maybe I needed to adjust my habits to fit into hers a little more. Then my mind wandered farther. I did know a few things about Mom. I knew she started her family very early in life, graduating high school pregnant and the salutatorian of her class. She married and had four more children, raising them with Joe's father until they divorced when Joe, the baby of the five, was nine. From then on, she raised those children on her own. She worked full time at Pratt & Whitney, sometimes working multiple jobs just to make ends meet.

I thought about the mind this woman must have. She was smart, maybe even brilliant. Without a college education she was a technical writer for Pratt & Whitney aircraft engines, the only woman in the department. In the house, there she sat working at one of the most prestigious crossword puzzles produced, this was what her Sunday down time was. This was where she found joy.

Me: So, let your Mom do her puzzle?
Joe: Yep.
Me: Don't ask her if she needs another cup of coffee?
Joe: Nope.
Me: Do you want an egg or pancakes? I can just make extra and let her know that it's there if she wants some.
Joe: Nah.
Me: Too much?
Joe: Yep.
Me: (sighing) I'm just trying.
Joe: (rubbing my arm) Come on, let's take a ride up to the bakery and see Joe and Joan for an egg sandwich.

Joe picked up the coffee mugs and brought them into the kitchen through the back door, closing it without it slamming. I walked around the side of the house and peeked through the dining room window. There was Mom, in exactly the same position, newspaper folded close to her face, concentrating hard.

Then I saw it. She pulled the paper down to the arm of the chair, a smile creeped across her face as she wrote on the paper. She reached across the arm and picked up her coffee and sipped it with her eyes closed for a moment. She returned the cup to the table, picked up the paper again, and stared hard at the puzzle. This was her time; she didn't need a chatty daughter-in-law disrupting her. As I stood watching this brilliant woman's mind work, I could have never known what a treasure I would find it to be more than twenty years later.

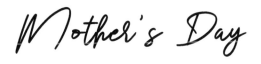

Mother's Day

Connecticut

May 2018

Mom sat in the dining hall with an intense look on her face. In one hand she held a spoon, the other a knife. She looked at the spoon and cautiously brought it to the pumpkin pie. She hesitated and pulled the spoon back and brought the knife closer. Mom let out a deep sigh and put the knife and spoon down, then blew her nose in her bib.

Me: How's dinner taste, Ma?
MIL: Hhmmmm?
Me: Dinner, how is it?
MIL: Good, I guess.
Me: Well, you're a gal after my own heart, going after that pie before you've eaten your dinner!
MIL: Oh yeah?
Me: (giggling) Yeah! I think we need to open a restaurant; we'll call it Dessert First!
MIL: Ummm, good idea?

Across the table Dorothy, another Star Unit resident, started chattering.

Dorothy: So nice of you to come today.
Joe: Glad we did.

Dorothy: Ya know you don't have to knock, you can just come right in.

Me: Really, how about one knock?

Dorothy: Well, one knock…okay. The weather's nice today, not so bad.

Joe: Sure is! It's a special day.

Dorothy: Yeah, well you can come by anytime, just come right in.

Joe: We'll do that.

Dorothy: I'm glad you came, it's a good day, nice day…yeah you come anytime.
    Don't worry about knocking just come right in.

I smiled across the table and Dorothy grinned ear to ear. Joe continued the banter back and forth with Dorothy, who was a chatter box that day. I returned my attention to Mom, who had quickly lost interest in Dorothy and had returned to the pie. She was diligently attacking it, with her spoon turned in the wrong direction so it was just slipping off the pie. Mom sighed again, although I noticed she didn't seem angry; frustrated a bit maybe, but not angry.

Me: Pie's looking good, Ma! Do you need help?

Joe: Here…

Joe leaned over and gently took the spoon from Mom. He scooped a piece of it and handed the spoon back to her.

Joe: They're tricky buggers, aren't they?

MIL: Who?

Joe: The spoon…

MIL: Oh yeah…(smiling weakly).

Dorothy, who was still chatting non-stop about not needing to knock when we visit, just to let ourselves in, stopped short in her sentence and gazed at Joe.

Dorothy: That's a good boy.

MIL: He sure is, and he's all mine.

Me: Hey, Beautiful! You gonna share him?

MIL: Well, just a little (smiling).

Me: Gosh, I hope so!

MIL: Easy, I said a little.

Joe smirked at me and chuckled. Dorothy smiled and lifted her glass of juice toward Joe.

Dorothy: Hey, have a beverage…it's a good beverage, you can have some, don't worry it's okay, its good. Yeah, good beverage, I'll leave it here for you…because it's a good beverage.

I think *Beverage, that's a big word*, and it rolls right off Dorothy's tongue. This disease is so unpredictable.

Joe looked over at Mom who was now just pushing food around on her plate.

Joe: You done, Mom?
MIL: Ummmm…(looking down on a plate that is half full), I think so…
Me: No pressure to eat everything on your plate. I mean, you ate the good stuff, the pie's gone!
MIL: Well, that was very good.
Joe: How about we clean up and head back to your room?
MIL: Yeah, good…

As we collected her things, Joe passed a small photo album and the remote for her TV to me. I was a little puzzled, Joe shrugged and returned to Mom.

Joe: Here we go.
MIL: Okay…where are we going?
Joe: Back to your room.
MIL: Oh, good.
Me: (whispering in Joe's ear) The TV remote?
Joe: (chuckling) I just want to know how she managed the walker, TV remote, and photo book in one trip?!
Me: (giggling) Well, when she's determined, she can move mountains.
MIL: What?
Me: Nothing, Beautiful. I was just telling Joe how much I admire your determination and grit!
MIL: (smiling and shaking her hip just a bit) Why, thank you!
Me: Come on, follow me. Can you follow exactly like me?

I walked a little like a duck and watched as other residents smiled and watched.

MIL: Yeah, noooooo (smiling and shaking her head).

I turned back and looked for Joe.

Joe: See ya later, Dorothy.
Dorothy: Ya, you come by no, need to knock, you just come on in…it'll be nice, kinda like today, it's a nice day to visit, just come in don't knock.
Joe: I will. We'll see you soon.
Dorothy: Yeah, just stop in.

We settled Mom into her room. I straightened a few things out. We were just here the evening before, so things were still in their proper place. Her room-mate Christine's cards and clothes weren't in her top drawer, and all the photos on her dresser were indeed hers. Mom often would do her own "straightening," moving her roommate Christine's photos to her dresser or stuffing her cards in the nightstand. I placed the flowers we brought for Mother's Day on her dresser.

Me: Whadya think, Beautiful? Pretty aren't they?
MIL: Yep.
Me: Joe picked them out. I like the different colors (spinning the pot of flowers for effect).
MIL: Me, too.

We settled her into bed. Joe sat in a chair next to her bed and I on her bed. Mom reached out and held our hands.

MIL: Thank you. I'm so glad you're here.
Me: I'm glad, too.
MIL: You're so good to me.
Me: You're good to us.
MIL: (smiling) Okay.

Mom closed her eyes. We watched the Hallmark Channel for a bit as she drifted off to sleep. I looked at Joe, he was watching her. We made eye contact and had our secret little exchange that said it was time to head out and let her rest.

Joe: (gently rubbing Mom's arm) Mom?
MIL: Hhhhmmm?
Joe: We're heading out.
MIL: Okay.
Me: I love you, Mom.

Mom opened her eyes. She smiled gently and warmly. Maybe I allowed my mind to play tricks on me, but I thought I saw her, really saw her.

MIL: I love you, too.

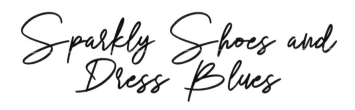

Sparkly Shoes and Dress Blues

Connecticut

October 2018

My niece Anna sat on my knee as I cut up her ham. Her little head brushed under my chin, the sensation tickled as much as it was pleasant. I pulled my chin back tight into my neck and kissed the top of her head.

Anna: Hey! (craning her head back and looking up at me)
Me: Hey what?
Anna: What dat you do?
Me: (giggling and squeezing her tighter) Do? I kissed your head!
Anna: (smiling wide, showing off a little chewed ham in her mouth) Why?
Me: 'Cause you make me happy!

She nestled her head into my chest a little closer, then shot her head back and giggled. I covered her forehead with more loving kisses. I couldn't resist that pint-sized round face, the sweet little voice, or the pure innocence that sat before me in this beautiful little being.

Anna: More pease!
Me: More? Look at you eatin' up all that ham! Here, I'll cut some of mine.
Anna: Tank you.

As I pulled the knife through the remaining ham on my plate, Anna rested her head on my right arm. She felt so good in my lap. I was desperately trying to stay in the moment and just enjoy this little treasure. However, as I cut, my mind wandered. I rolled out my checklist in my head and absent-mindedly glanced at my watch, 12:45 p.m.

Me: Joe?

Holding onto Anna's precious little bottom and thigh, I turned in my seat to face the family room.

Me: Honey?
Joe: Yes, dear?

Joe smirked and turned toward me. He knew how much I hated it when he said, "Yes, dear."

Me: I'm thinking we leave here by 2:45? We should get ready before we visit your Mom.
Joe: Why don't we just swing by and see her first?
Me: Drive to Wallingford and back? Then back to Wallingford?
Joe: Yeah, that way we're not all dressed up when we go.

I processed the timing. I also was already planning out the visit with Mom. It had become part of my routine of late to think through what we would talk about when we visited. I was coming up short on ideas, but that day I thought if we arrived dressed, well there would be plenty to talk about.

Me: No...let's go dressed. I need too much time to plaster and spackle this face of mine.
Anna: (looking confused) Paster and speckle you face?
Me: (smiling and chuckling lightly) It means I need a lot of time to put on my make-up and do my hair.

Penny, my other niece, Anna's sister, was sitting on the bench next to us and was now very interested in our conversation.

Penny: You gonna wear a pretty dress?

Anna: Ohhh petty dress?

Me: Yep! And sparkly shoes. I love sparkly shoes!

Penny: Meeee too!!

Anna: (bouncing on my knee) Me too! Me too! Me too!

Me: (leaning close to both their heads and whispering) Sparkly shoes always make me feel so pretty. Don't you think so?

Two sets of wide eyes looked up at me as I continued to talk about how handsome their Uncle Joe would look in his dress blues, and how I would spend a little extra time on my hair and not forget my very glittery eye shadow. You would have thought I was talking about transforming into Cinderella herself.

I spent the next few hours trying to stay focused on my family, the precious gifts that surrounded me, my sisters and their husbands, my nieces and nephews, and my parents, who I thank God every day are in such good health. I colored with Penny, sat with my dad for a few minutes talking about a recent trip to North Carolina, and held my Mom just a little tighter when I thanked her for making dinner for us.

I went and found Joe, who was intently watching the Patriots game, and placed my hand on his shoulder.

Me: Hey, you ready?

Joe: Yea, I guess. Are you sure we shouldn't just stop by my mother's first?

Me: It's far too late now. I need time, ya know, for all of this (waving my hand over my face and guiding it over my body). This takes a lot longer than it used to.

Joe: (shaking his head and rolling his eyes) You're beautiful, you don't need any of...

Me: (cutting him off) Thanks, but I do. Let's go.

I did, indeed, need the time, but we cleaned up nicely, if I did say so myself. As we walked into Regency House, I knew my gut was right. My thought that our fancy attire would please the residents was spot on. Gathered in the front room were residents with a few family members just visiting. This was a generation who loved to dress, who took pride in how they looked and always appreciated a man in uniform. We were glamorous, Joe in his dress blues and I in a long black coat with an amber and gold fur collar that filled my shoulders. The residents showered us with compliments as we hammed it up a bit, walking like we were on the red carpet through the lobby.

Me: (giggling) Oh, they are fun.
Joe: (shaking his head) You're nuts.
Me: I am (winking). Wait 'til we get to Mom's unit.

We made our way down the hall. As I waited for Joe to punch the code into the keypad, I peeked through the safety glass at Mom who sat in the dining room staring directly at me. I waved and watched her eyes dart from left to right. She had no idea who I was.

Joe: Here we go (pushing the door open and allowing me to pass).
Me: She's in the dining room.
Joe: I saw.

I took a deep breath and smiled widely, feeling my eyes start to dance. I spun to the right and entered the dining room, walking tall and regal with Joe close on my heels. An aide was the first to notice us as we entered.

Aide: Wellllll, look at this!? Wowza! Girllll, you look great!
Me: (pausing to strike a quick red carpet pose) Why, thank you. We're off to
    a ball this evening!

I made my way to Mom's table, listening to the aides and residents chatter about how beautiful we looked. I stopped about five feet from Mom's chair and paused. She had heard the commotion and was studying me carefully. I knew she had no idea who I was. I felt that familiar twinge of disappointment that she didn't know me. After all this time, you would think I'd just come to expect it, but I just couldn't. I blinked away the feeling and concentrated on making sure my eyes were dancing and the energy I was putting out was positive.

Me: Well, hello there, Beautiful. How's my girl?
MIL: Hi?
Me: (pointing over Mom's shoulder at Joe) Look who I have with me!

MIL: (turning to look and startled to see Joe) Oh? Hello!

Me: (leaning in a little) Doesn't he look so handsome?!

MIL: (looking him up and down) Uh huh!

Joe: Hi, Ma (leaning down and kissing her forehead).

Aide: Wow, you two look amazing!

MIL: (looking up at me, still no recollection of who I am) Yes, you look nice!

Me: Thanks, Ma! I thought you'd like to see us all gussied up!

I leaned down and kissed her, leaving a perfect red kiss mark on her cheek.

Me: Dang it (wiping gently at her cheek), I got lipstick on you!

Doris: Feurb me shas! Feurb...

Aide: Doris likes your shoes.

Doris was another resident at Regency House. I worked hard each time I saw Doris to understand her, I never did. I know she got frustrated with me, I got frustrated with me, too. I turned on my heel and pulled up the hem of my dress, twisting my ankle a little to allow the light to catch the strap of sequins that dressed my ankle.

Doris: WOW...

That I understood.

Me: You like them?

Doris: Uh huh!

MIL: (leaning down for a closer look herself) Ohhhh, that's nice...

Dorothy: Yes, that's very nice, very fancy, you look so good. You should stop by more often, yes, just come in, in that...yes fancy.

Me: (giggling a little) Thanks, Dorothy! You like my outfit? Did you see Joe? He's mighty dapper too!

Dorothy: Oh yes, so handsome, so nice...

MIL: Uh huh

Joe: Honey? Christine is watching you (pointing behind me over my shoulder).

Me: (turning to wave to her) I'll be right back. I'm going to say hi.

I approached Christine's table, she was smiling and holding her hand out to me. This woman, who I'd only known since January, was reaching for me, knew who I was, but my own mother-in-law of twenty-eight years couldn't connect with me. My heart hurt, yet I pushed the feeling aside. I reached toward Christine.

Christine: Ohhhhhh…

Me: Hello, Christine (holding one hand and lightly stroking her shoulder), how are you?

Christine: Goooood (smiling and watching me as if she's a little star struck), gooood.

Me: It's so good to see you! You look wonderful today.

Christine: (smiling) Ahhhhh (stroking the side of my coat).

Me: Nice, isn't it? (leaning down so my fur collar is closer to her). I always feel so graceful in this coat, feel the collar.

Christine reached up, never taking her eyes off my face, and stroked the collar. I let her enjoy the soft texture and glamour of the coat. I spent a few minutes with her and the other residents sharing her dining table, then excused myself to return to Mom's table.

I walked toward the table, watching Joe cutting Mom's meatloaf. She sat hunched over, staring at her plate, hands on her lap as Joe prepped her plate. Dorothy chatted behind him about visiting again and us being "fancy." It was probably silly, but that warmed my heart. I stood between Mom and Doris, attempting small talk with Mom.

Doris: Fud pease (pushing her meatloaf with a spoon).

Me: …and we'll be at the Oakdale, is that what they're calling it now or is it sponsored by someone?

Joe: It's the Oakdale.

Doris: FUD, pease.

Joe: Doris? Do you need help?

Doris: Yeah hhh…

Me: Do you need me to cut that for you?

Doris: Uh huh (looking up with her chin dropped open and her tongue slightly extended).

Me: I'll help…

I assessed the position of her wheelchair, which was backed against our favorite resident marine's wheelchair. I realized I couldn't get around the two chairs, so I cautiously leaned in around Doris.

Me: Doris, I'm going to cut this up okay?

In the past, probably out of frustration, Doris had had a few outbursts that I'd witnessed. I wasn't sure how she would react to my leaning over her to cut the meatloaf.

Doris: Ohhhhhh kayyyyy…

Slowly I cut her meatloaf, talking quietly as I did so. My right arm over her right shoulder, my left over her left side. As I cut, she leaned her head on my right arm, her eyes were closed, and a faint smile crossed her face. I flashed back to earlier in the day when Anna sat on my lap as I cut her ham. I hardly knew Doris, yet my heart was sad. What I saw before me was a woman who craved human touch, a loving gesture, and maybe a feeling of being special for a moment. I looked over to Mom who was trying to scoop up her meatloaf with a knife, Joe was already picking up the fork and handing it to her.

Me: Mom?

MIL: (looking up at me blankly) Huh?

Me: How's your dinner?

MIL: Good.

I finished cutting Doris's dinner and gave her shoulder a squeeze. She mumbled something that sounded like a thank you as I directed my attention to Mom.

Me: So, honestly, is the meatloaf better than mine?

MIL: Yeah.

Me: (making a buzzing sound) Wrong answer! You love my meatloaf!

MIL: If you say so (rolling her eyes).

Me: (giggling) I do say so! Joe's not a huge fan (winking at Joe).

Now I was scrambling for conversation starters.

Joe: Your meatloaf is okay.
MIL: Yeah, what he said.
Me: Hey!

Mom looked up at me and for a moment I thought I saw some depth in her eyes, like she was possibly going to make a connection, but it was gone as fast as it arrived. That awkward silence fell over the table. Joe stood on Mom's left, I on her right, and we watched her eat. I scrambled in my head for what we could talk about while Joe intercepted a new resident on Mom's left from drinking Mom's juice.

Me: Good catch (smiling at Joe).
Joe: Here, Ma, drink up.
MIL: Uh huh.

Mom pushed the food around on her plate. She had eaten well but had lost interest in what was left. Joe pulled her walker closer so we could return to her room. Once again, as we made our way through the dining hall, all eyes were on us. Dorothy reminded us to come back and visit soon. We didn't have to knock. Christine waved and watched us adoringly. Our favorite marine even smiled as we passed. We settled Mom into her room. I showered her with love and kisses. Me having to once again wipe lipstick off her cheek did get a playful response from her, which made my heart happy for a moment.

Then it was time for us to go. We said our goodbyes. Walking through the lobby we, once again, received compliments and kudos for our glamorous attire. As the sliding doors opened, I smiled and waved goodbye to the residents and turned back to Joe.

Me: Yep, going dressed was a good idea.
Joe: It was.
Me: Who doesn't love seeing sparkly shoes and dress blues?

Joe: (shaking his head and smiling) Yeah.
Me: They loved it, and not only in Mom's unit!

Joe kissed my cheek and opened the car door for me. As I turned to step into the car the sun caught his badge. A wave of loss flowed over me. Mom wouldn't remember this day, she wouldn't remember how handsome Joe was, and that made my heart ache. She would have been so proud of her son. I made a note to myself to talk about today and how amazing her son is the next time I visit. I looked down to my feet and adjusted that sparkly strap on my shoes, they were a good choice for tonight's visit.

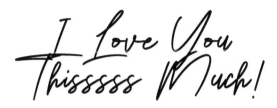

Connecticut

October 2018

My black leather pump applied pressure to the brake as my right hand sat on the gear shift, which was securely in park. I was exhausted, energized, and apprehensive all rolled into one emotional state. I had worked more than forty hours for the week already and it was only Wednesday afternoon, so my exhaustion was warranted. I was energized because my team and I had a 7:00 a.m. presentation that morning that was wildly successful. We were well on our way to designing an amazing project with dream clients. If that wasn't enough of a rollercoaster of emotions, I now sat, apprehensive, with my foot still on the brake, uncertain of what I would find today with Mom. I sat for a moment longer, then rolled my shoulders to attempt to release some stress and checked my reflection in the rearview mirror. I was pleasantly surprised my eyes weren't completely bloodshot from lack of sleep. I didn't tend to visit Mom in the middle of the afternoon, Joe usually did. We often received calls and reports from the staff that afternoons were difficult times for her, Joe had experienced it, too. We had learned that Alzheimer's patients sometimes experience "sundowning," where their difficult times come as the sun sets. We had discovered that while the sun setting did affect Mom, she additionally had the afternoons to contend with.

I heard the lock click as I finished punching the code into the keypad outside Mom's unit. I firmly placed my palm on the door, pushing it open. I switched the gears in my head as I stepped through the door. Any apprehension I might have been harboring at the present needed to be tabled, there was no room for any of it right then. As I closed the door behind me, Yolanda, the head nurse, rounded the corner wearing a bright smile.

Yolanda: Hey Girl! What you doin' here in the middle of the day?
Me: I have a CEU tonight, and a trip in the morning. So, how is she this afternoon?
Yolanda: (shrugging her shoulder a bit, tilting her head toward the end of the hall) She's okay?

The question at the end of her sentence didn't instill any confidence in me. Still, I knew better than to predetermine how my visit would go, I knew I set the tone.

Me: Well, let's see if we can't make her a little happier.
Yolanda: Girl, if anyone can…

Yolanda turned quickly at a sudden repetitive banging around the corner. She flashes me a warm smile of encouragement, turned, and headed in the direction of the banging.

Yolanda: Henry? Oh, Henry, here I got that…where you goin'?

I stepped by the doorway to see Yolanda carefully redirecting Henry in his wheelchair. Clearly, he had been running his chair directly into the wall of his room. Her hand gently stroked his arm as she spoke gently and softly to him. He looked blankly at her, his jaw dropped wide open while grunts escaped his throat.

I always found great comfort in seeing the staff treat the residents with such kindness and compassion. I continued down the hall to find Mom sitting by herself in a chair at the end of the hallway. I could already see the scowl on her face. I did a quick pep talk with myself, reminding myself, again, that I was in control of the direction our visit would take.

Me: Hey there, Mom!

Nothing, not even a turn of the head in my direction. I stepped closer, now I was right at her side.

Me: Hey there, Beautiful!

I placed my hand carefully on her arm. She jumped and pulled her arm away abruptly. Her eyebrows were knitted tightly together, but her eyes didn't project fear; they were brewing anger and rage. I forced a smile, hoping and silently praying she would feel the love and tenderness I was projecting.

Me: How are you?
MIL: (staring at me with laser eyes) Goooood?
Me: (placing my hand on her shoulder and giving it a gentle squeeze) You look fabulous!
MIL: (pulling away from my touch) Oh…

Mom turned her head away from me and I thought, *I am far too tired for this.* I watched her for a moment, staring at the wall as I rubbed the back of my neck attempting to loosen the knot that was growing. Mom turned her head slightly and looked at me out of the corner of her eyes. The corner of her lip curled up. I pulled a chair closer to hers and sat.

Me: So, it's a beautiful day, do you see…
MIL: (slightly screeching) What do you want?!
Me: I'd like to visit with you.
MIL: No.
Me: No?
MIL: I know you…

Mom leaned in close to me, her eyes sending a message of distrust. I am not deterred.

Me: Of course, you know me, I'm your…
MIL: Yeah…you . . you…

Mom slammed her hand on the arm of the chair and turned away.

Me: Mom? (cautiously laying my hand on her arm again)
MIL: Don't…don't you…GET! (voice rising). You think…you think yourrrr
    so…GET!

I pulled back. It has been months since I'd experienced this level of anger and
frustration from her. My overtired mind scrambled for ideas on how to dif-
fuse this before it escalated out of control. I knew she thought I was there to
take whomever she believed was her man. Those days, Mom flipped between
remembering her ex-husband and remembering Fred. I didn't know who she
thought I was there to take from her, nevertheless I had become a threat.

Me: How about I just sit with you for a few minutes? I don't have to talk; I
    can just be with you.
MIL: No.
Me: (sighing) Well…you might not like me very much right now, but I love
    you and want to spend time with you.
MIL: I don't care…GO!

My eyes started to burn. They didn't burn from lack of sleep, they burned
because tears were quickly brewing. I looked up and saw Yolanda watching us
carefully. I smiled weakly and nodded toward her, indicating we were okay.
I decided to just sit for a spell, collect myself, and figure out how to turn the
visit around.

MIL: Humph (fidgeting in her chair).
Me: Need something, Beautiful?
MIL: Don't call me that! (folding her arms tightly across her chest)
Me: Well, you happen to be one of the most beautiful women I know.
MIL: (eyes darting left to right) Yeah, right.

Mom turned to focus on me, fury still filling her eyes.

Me: (cautiously) I speak the truth, you are beautiful.
MIL: Huh? (looking at me cautiously)
Me: Yep, you're an amazing woman, one I admire.

MIL: You what? Ad...ameeer...huh? (her face softening)

I thought, *Here we go, we're turning the corner.*

Me: Admire...I admire you!
MIL: You...you do?
Me: (leaning a little closer) Yes, you are smart, you are beautiful, you are a
    wonderful mom and grandma, but most importantly you are very, very
    important to me.

She studied me for a moment.

MIL: I...I...(sighing)
Me: (kissing her cheek and lightly touching my forehead to hers) I love
    you, Mom.

She leaned back. I looked squarely into her eyes. It was gone, the anger was
gone. She looked down at her hands and back up at me.

MIL: I...you...(confusion crossing her face) you...I don't...

Mom made eye contact with me and she looked so sad it made my heart hurt.

Me: Shhh. It's going to be okay.
MIL: (sighing deeply and looking up to the ceiling) Is it?
Me: Heck yeah!
MIL: Oh?
Me: Yep, 'cause we've got love, and love fixes everything.
MIL: Oh?

I started scrambling for something to connect this, to explain how love fixes
everything and keep this momentum going. I fell back on an old standby—my
kids. Stories of my babies almost always made Mom smile.

Me: Yep, love fixes everything; it wins every time. You always loved the way
    my little Joey would say "I love you"!
MIL: Did I?

Me: When Joey was little, you lived with us for a while. You had been very sick and needed some help during your recovery.

MIL: Oh? I don't re...re...(tapping her forehead) I...I don't reeee (sighing) remem...member...

Me: How about I help you remember (smiling and opening my eyes wide with excitement). I'm sure you'll like the memory.

MIL: Yeah, do that...

I leaned back in my chair and took her down Memory Lane. I took Mom back to 2001 when she lived with us while recovering from necrotizing fasciitis. During her stay, my sitting room became her bedroom. There was never a door on the room, so for privacy I had hung a simple curtain. Mom was never a morning person, and well, we are, so mornings were tough for her in our house.

Me: Oh, you were patient, Mom! Joey was always so excited to see you in the morning that he'd plant his face against the curtain and whisper/yell...

I leaned in a little closer to Mom for effect and explained what it meant to whisper/yell.

Me: That's when you try to speak really loudly but you're still whispering.

MIL: (smiling) Oh yeah?

Me: Yes, he'd whisper/yell with his face against the curtain (holding my hand in front of my face like it was a curtain) "GAMMA?!...GAMMA?!...You AWAKE?" (giggling). I'd scoop him up, which was difficult he was three and the size of a five-year-old! I'd pull him away from the curtain and explain you were sleeping, and that you needed your beauty rest.

MIL: Uh huh...

Me: I don't know how he would do it, but most mornings I'd turn my back for only a moment and he'd be gone! Do you know where he went?

MIL: No.

Me: He scooted behind the curtain and was standing at your bedside! Guess what he was doing?

MIL: (shaking her head, her eyes searching my face for an answer) What?

Me: Standing over your bed whisper/yelling "GAMMA?!...GAMMA?!...You AWAKE?"

MIL: (starting to laugh) Really? Oh...

Me: Yep! I'd have to scoop him up again, most mornings you'd roll over and say it was okay, that you were up anyway (shaking my head). But really he had woken you up, you were never a morning person!

MIL: No?

Me: Nope! If you had it your way, you'd get up at the crack of noon!

MIL: Crack of what?

Me: Noon. But Joey had a way of waking you up and making you smile.

MIL: Oh?

Me: He was so darn cute. I'd usually lightly scold him for waking you up, but he always had the perfect response. Want to know what it was?

MIL: Yeah (a smile creeping across her face).

Me: (standing up) He'd say, "GAMMA? Don't be mad. I don't wake you for nuttin'! I wake you 'cause I love you thissssss much!"

I re-enacted Joey as a three-year-old stretching my arms so wide my hands touched behind my back.

Mom's head shot back and a hearty laugh escaped her lungs. She held her belly and let the happy memory and good feelings fill her soul. I soaked up the moment.

Yes, love wins, or at least it did that afternoon.

We sat for a spell longer before I settled her in the dining room for dinner. At her table Dorothy started chatting about how glad she was that I came for a visit. I stroked Mom's shoulder and kissed the top of her head.

Me: I'm going to head out, Mom. I love you.

MIL: I love you to (looking up at me, smiling warmly).

Me: Yep, love fixes everything, Mom.

MIL: It does?

Me: Trust me, Mom, it does.

MIL: Okay.

As I left the unit, I stopped outside the dining room to wave to Mom behind the glass window. She looked directly at me, actually through me, blankly. I blew her a kiss, more for me than for her, reminding myself love wins, every time.

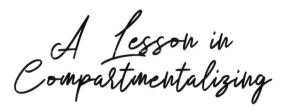

A Lesson in Compartmentalizing

Florida

November 2018

I sat in my client's great room in Florida discussing delivery schedules for their new home furnishings. Over my client's head was a clock showing me the time was already 11:15 a.m. That little wave of anxiety started to flutter in my chest, the one that arrives every time I'm winding down the work in one office to head to the next. I was mentally checking off the list of what I had accomplished and what I still needed to button up before my flight. I returned my focus to my client and compared their travel schedule with mine, dialing in on optimal delivery dates. I felt my Apple watch vibrate on my wrist. It's always a careful little dance I do as I try to glance at the text coming in but not lose focus on my client. I glanced and saw it was a text from Joe. Experience had taught me that important text messages are long, other text messages are one-liners. This one filled my screen. I knew instinctively it was something that needed my attention.

Me: My apologies (leaning toward my purse to grab my phone), this is Joe. I'd like to check my phone more closely to see what he needs.
Client: Oh, yes! Of course!!!

It was exactly the response I expected because I am blessed with an amazing clientele, every one of them adores my husband.

Me: Thanks, I know we're short on time.
Client: Psssshhh, don't be silly! We're just about done. We need to get you outta here and on a plane to Joe!

Before I started reading the text, I looked at both my clients and smiled, thanking God for blessing me with such understanding, amazing clients.

Text from Joe: Mom's leg has gotten bad again, two spots looking bad. Sue is coming to take a look. I'm pretty sure she has venous ulcers. It's when blood flow in the leg isn't good enough, leading to sores. Takes weeks to months to heal. No official diagnosis, but that's what I think.

A second wave of uneasiness filled my chest, tears stung the back of my eyes. I slid the phone into the side pocket of my purse. The guilt I felt when I was away from Connecticut could become overwhelming at times, especially when it came to Joe and Mom. Nevertheless, I needed to compartmentalize for a moment. I was running short on time, I could call Joe from the car.

Client: All good with Joe?
Me: Yeah, it's my mother in-law. I'll call him in a few.
Client: I'm sorry, I hope she's okay.

Just compartmentalize, I tell myself.

Me: Oh, yes, as well as she can be!

I smiled and looked away because that amazingly understanding client had reached over and gently squeezed my knee. I could feel the tears threatening again. It's always the words of kindness that break me. *Compartmentalize.*

I reviewed our agenda to ensure we'd covered all the important issues and made our next appointment. We shared warm hugs and well wishes as they walked me to the door.

Once at my car, I packed binders and samples into my front seat and quickly skipped around the front of the car to access the driver's side. As I opened my car door, I looked up to see my clients standing in the driveway smiling.

Client: Hey, Lisa?

Me: Yeah?

Client: Safe travels and get home to Joe. I'm sure your mother in law will be okay (blowing a kiss and waving).

Me: Thanks. You don't know how much I appreciate that.

Client: Go on now, get outta here!

I backed my car out of the driveway and, before I scooted away, I paused and looked out the passenger side window. My clients were waving well wishes from the driveway. I thought, *God sends me angels all the time.* These two angels somehow, unbeknownst to them, had calmed my soul.

By the time I reached the gate to leave, I had already started dialing Joe.

Joe: Hello?

Me: Hey, How's she doin'?

Joe: She's good.

Me: How bad is the leg?

Joe: Its not lookin' good.

Me: I thought we were on the mend?

Joe: Me too…huh? Yeah, no I'm waiting…uh huh…okay, yes that's important. She keeps reopening it…yep, yeah okay.

Me: Who's that?

Joe: Nurse, she's giving me some updates, they need to get Coban tape. She can't pull that off.

Me: I don't understand why this isn't healing?

Joe: It's hard honey…she…what? Okay…Ma, you ready for lunch?…Yes, hm-mumm (chuckling). Okay, that'll do. Sorry, Honey, what was I sayin'?

Me: We were talking about Mom's leg? Why doesn't it heal, why can't we fix this?

Joe: Honey, she's okay…it's complicated….Hey, Ma? It's Lisa, want to say hello?

Me: Yes! Let me say hello!

MIL: Helllllooo?

Me: (talking slowly and clearly) Heya, Beautiful!

MIL: Hiiiiii…

Me: I'm coming home tonight, Ma!

MIL: Huh?…I'm going home tonight?

Me: Me, Mom, me. *I'm* coming home tonight.

MIL: Oh!

Me: I miss (my voice cracking) you so much, Mom.

MIL: I miss you, too.

Me: I can't wait to wrap my arms around you…

MIL: Hhmmmm, yeah.…You make me feel good…

Me: *You* make *me* feel good, Ma!

MIL: (giggling) That's good!

Me: I love you!

MIL: Yeah.

Me: (chuckling) Okay, I'll see you tomorrow?

MIL: Okay…bye…

Joe: Hey?

Me: Wow, that went well!!!!

Joe: Yep, sure did.

The anxiety started to slip away. Even though there were miles between us, somehow his voice was as soothing as his touch, and his touch always has a calming effect.

Me: That's the best phone conversation I've had in a long time!

Joe: Yep…here ya go, Ma…Yep it was!…What? Yes, that'll work…sorry, Honey…

Me: It's okay. I'm stopping at the apartment, then the office, then to the airport.

Joe: You remember I'm working tonight, right?

Me: Yes. I love you.

Joe: Love you, too.

I pressed "end" on my dashboard and my mind began to wander. Those sores on Mom's leg were in the area her skin graft was placed after her necrotizing fasciitis. I remembered the months she lived with us. It was a challenging experience for all of us. Mom had fallen ill on Father's Day 2001. After months in a hospital in Boston, she was transferred to Connecticut for additional re-habilitation. When that phase of the rehab was completed, she was still not strong enough to make the trip back to Arkansas, where she was living at the time, so she moved in with Joe and me and the kids. I settled my head against the headrest and relived those days.

On Monday September 10, 2001, Joe entered paramedic school. On Tuesday, September 11, well I don't need to tell anyone what happened that day. On Wednesday, September 12, I picked Mom up at the rehabilitation center in a neighboring town to bring her home to live and rehab with us for what would turn out to be six months. At the time, Joey was three, and Ashley was nine. I was working full time, Joe was attending classes Monday, Wednesday, and Friday, 6:00 to 10:00 p.m. in Hartford, and also doing full-day clinicals on Saturday.

With everything we had going on, I'll admit I was a little over-whelmed when Joe floated the idea of Mom living with us while she finished her rehab. No, let's be honest, I looked at him like he had sprouted a third head. I think I may have even told him he was nuts! In the end, though, he had pulled at my heartstrings. He knew, and I knew, the best place for her was with us. Well, with Joe, really; I was just a support role. So, I agreed.

During those months, Mom and I built a very special bond. What I didn't know, was that Mom thought I was that "perfect wife and mother." I could cook, I kept a fairly neat house, I ran a strict household—no television during the week, eating dinner as a family, only two extracurricular activities at one time, no PG movies until you were twelve—yeah, somehow she thought I was "perfect."

Then it happened. One night when Joe was in school, I ruined dinner, I forgot to wash Ashley's Brownie uniform, and I failed at the potty training with Joey. I collapsed on the sofa next to Mom and sighed heavily.

MIL: You okay?
Me: Meh.
MIL: You sure?
Me: I…I don't…(sniffling) I don't know, Ma.
MIL: What don't you know?
Me: Sometimes…well…sometimes it's a little much.
MIL: Hmmmm, yeah; I'd imagine so.
Me: I'm okay…Really, I am…sometimes I just need to (gulping)…
MIL: Need what?
Me: I don't know…

A tear escaped and slid down my cheek.

MIL: Tell me.
Me: I don't know if I can keep doing it…Joe is gone three nights a week and all day on Saturday…all he does is study when he is home. He's exhausted from working and studying (sniffling). Joey is a handful…why isn't he using the potty? I mean…how hard is it to aim at the damn freaking cheerios?! I feel like I don't give enough to Ashley…she's such a huge help, still I yell and scream at her for no reason…and tonight…ugh…dinner was disaster!!! I can't believe you choked that God awful mess from the crock pot down your throat! And have you seen me lately? (grabbing the part of my hair and pulling it apart) Look at these rooooots! My GAWD, I look like a train wreck!

Mom pulled her head back and opened her eyes wide. I blinked back tears as a I watched a smirk creep across her face.

MIL: That's it?
Me: (stunned) What?
MIL: That's it? (laughing lightly) That's all you got? You got this.

Me: No! I don't…I didn't even tell you about work! I mistakenly ordered the wrong hand-printed wallpaper at the cost of $1,200.00…I completely forgot an appointment to measure a backsplash and I have a presentation next week…shit…I don't even know how I'm going to make the project work, the client is asking for the impossible!

MIL: Yep, ya do. You got it (still smirking).

A tear slipped down my cheek. I looked at Mom as her eyes became intense, and that smirk softened into a warm smile. She opened her arms to me, and I collapsed into them and just cried. I cried big sobs that make you snort and gasp for air. She stroked my back and comforted me. I don't know how, but the next thing I knew the 11:00 p.m. news was blasting out of the television speakers and Mom was gently stroking my head. I had fallen asleep in her lap. I turned and looked up at her. The tears were dried from my cheeks, and I was a little, to say the least, embarrassed about my little hissy fit.

Me: Mom?

MIL: Hhhhmmmm?

Me: I'm sorry…

MIL: What for?

Me: (sitting up and letting out a little snort) Ummm, were you in the same room where I had that massive break down?

MIL: That? Pssshhh, that's nothing. I actually liked seeing you not so perfect (chuckling).

Me: Perfect?! Ma?! I'm far from perfect!

Mom was silent for a moment.

MIL: I'm sorry I'm such a burden.

Me: What? Oh my GOD! No!

Tears stung my eyes again, they always hurt even more when they return after a good cry!

Me: Mom...no. You. Are. Not. A. Burden....Please don't ever think that.

MIL: You have to admit, it would be easier if you didn't have to add me and all my (waving her hand over her bandaged legs) needs to your list of things to do.

I looked at Mom and sighed. Yes, it was a lot to juggle doctor appointments, dressing changes, visiting nurses' schedules, and medications with everything else that was going on, and honestly, I have my own Mom who I can run to, cry with, be comforted by. I knew she would tell me I'm doing a great, we'd make it just fine, etc. But at that moment, I looked at the woman in front of me and had a moment of clarity that I thank God for every day. She had given me the greatest gift I could have ever received second only to my babies. She gave me her son. I owed her.

Me: Ma?
MIL: (looking down into her lap) Yeah?
Me: Ma, look at me.

She raised her head and made direct eye contact with me.

Me: I couldn't do this without YOU!
MIL: Huh?
Me: Mom, you're a pillar of strength for me right now. I love coming home and calling out to you and hearing you yell back. My babies can't wait to see you when I pull into the driveway. I swear, seat belts are flying before I'm halfway up the driveway. You make me smile, you remind me daily I can get through this unbelievable journey Joe and I have decided we could navigate. Where would I be right now if you were home in Arkansas? I'd be alone on this sofa, crying, having a hissy fit while Joe was in class. He'd walk through the door and I'd probably yell at him for something stupid.
MIL: No you wouldn't
Me: Hell ya, I would!

MIL: (starting to laugh) No.
Me: Look at me. You're an inspiration to me. Sometimes I look at you and can't believe what you've accomplished in life.
MIL: Well, thank you, but...
Me: But nothing.

The back door opened. I heard Sophie, our dog, greet Joe with that unwavering devotion and love that all good dogs possess.

Joe: Hellllo?
Me: Hey!
MIL: Hello!

Joe entered the family room and could tell, after eleven years of marriage, immediately that I'd had a rough night. Well, maybe the bright red nose and puffy eyes gave it away.

Joe: All okay?
MIL: Yep, we are great. How was class?
Joe: Good?
MIL: Good.

Mom rubbed my shoulder, then gave me a light tap. She looked up at Joe and smiled. She asked some random questions about his class and the traffic coming home, but I honestly don't remember what. I do remember how she refocused the conversation so I could compartmentalize my night. So I could put away my feelings of being overwhelmed, of not being "perfect," of not being good enough. Mom knew exactly what she was doing at the moment. What she didn't know was that she was teaching me how to accept and live our journey ten-plus years in the future. I watched intently as Joe explained what he had learned in class to her, and how excited he was about Saturday's clinicals at the hospital. I realized God knew exactly what he was doing.

I turned the corner onto Pine Ridge Road where the apartment was located. That important checklist in my head pushed away the beautiful memory. Turn down the air, take out the garbage, wipe down counters, double check the dryer, don't forget to water the lime tree…Joe will love the limes next month.

As I turned into the entry to my apartment building, a tear hit the steering wheel. I wiped my cheek and put the car in park. I put my head back against the headrest and remember the woman who helped guide me through a very challenging chapter of my life. I had people tell me that I'm a saint for what I do for my mother-in-law. I'm no saint, I'm just returning the favor.

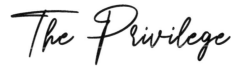

The Privilege

Connecticut

November 2018

It was 7:40 p.m. I fell onto the sofa and opened my laptop. I scanned my emails, answered one pressing issue, smiled as I read through an email from a client sending praise for my hardworking team, and closed out that tab in the browser. As I did every day, I typed "Face" into the empty browser search bar, quickly pulling up my Facebook account. The first post that popped up in my feed was a photo of my beautiful daughter. The photo was cropped, so I could only see her chin, neck, ear, and flowing blonde hair. I would know that face anywhere. My heart swelled in my chest. Funny, she was twenty-six years old and I still wanted to climb into my computer and kiss that lovely cheek. I smiled and scrolled to read her post.

A few years ago, while she was still having longer lucid moments, my grandmother gifted me the bulk of her jewelry collection. All the pieces were so unique, so utterly expressive of who she was as a person. For a long time, it hurt my heart to wear them. They were a constant reminder of the vibrant person she was— a person I miss deep down in my bones. I wear her jewelry now, and I've started to add my own meaningful pieces to her (our) collection like these from A Tea Leaf Jewelry. I cherish the privilege of

keeping her strong spirit alive. #heirloomjewelry #lifewithmil #alzheimers

I paused, sipped my glass of wine, and then my mind took off like a bullet out of the chamber of a gun. The memories flooded in, and I landed in my kitchen six years ago.

Joe: Mom's going to need cardiac rehab.
Me: (leaning against the kitchen counter reaching for the steaming cup Joe was handing me) Cardiac rehab, what does that entail?
Joe: (slurping) Visits to the rehab center a couple times a week.

Ashley stumbled into the kitchen, her platinum blonde hair tussled from a night of great slumber. She stopped at the edge of the counter, stretched her arms tall and wide, and let an obnoxious yawn escape her mouth.

Ashley: (smacking her lips, dismissing the yawn) Morning! Whoa!

Ashley caught her balance as Izzy, our one-hundred-pound Rottweiler, greeted her by pushing her robust, powerful frame between Ashley's legs. I smiled as I watched the morning ritual start to unfold. Ashley giggled as she scratched Izzy's body, the dogs tail shook so hard with excitement that Ashley had to steady herself with one hand on the wall.

Joe: Morning, Baby! Easy, Izzy! (leaning down and rubbing the dogs big loving head)
Me: Morning.

I was now completely preoccupied with this latest news about rehab.

Ashley: (pouring coffee into a mug and adding a heaping spoonful of sugar) What's this rehab stuff you're all talking about?

Me: Easy with the sugar, Baby.

Ashley: (rolling her eyes) Yes, Mommmmmm.

Joe: Grandma needs cardiac rehab.

Ashley: What is that?

Joe: Well, it happens at a rehab facility, she will walk on a treadmill, probably do other exercises to raise her heart rate and they'll monitor her.

Me: How often? I'm worried about getting her there, I've already got two days lost this month with the Yale study, work is insane, plus getting Joey around to boy scouts and...

Joe: I could ask my brothers to pitch in...

I looked at Joe, his brothers were great, our sisters-in-law, too. But it was always a challenge when we needed help with Mom. Part of it was distance, we were three miles from her house while they ranged from forty-five minutes to an hour away. The other reason was that they had a little less flexibility in their schedules and careers.

Ashley: Mama?

Me: (sipping the coffee) Hmmmm?

Ashley: I can help.

Me: Oh, Baby, thank you, but you have school.

Ashley: Well, we'll work her appointments around my classes. As long as you can spare me at the studio...

Joe: Grandma's not going to like going, she could get a little tough.

Me: I don't know (looking at Joe), maybe I can work something out between your days off and my schedule. When's the first appointment?

Joe: Today. I'm going to take her and get her settled and understand the schedule.

Me: Okay, send me wha...

Ashley: Daddy, let me get my schedule for class, that way you can work it around the classes. It will just work better this way (now yelling across the house as she retrieved her schedule). I'll be fine with Grandma, we share a birthday for crying out loud! (coming back into the kitchen and placing her schedule on the counter in front of Joe) She can't get mad at me, I was the ultimate birthday gift! (turning on her heel and rounding the corner into the hallway) Getting in the shower!!!!

I looked up at Joe, he was watching the now empty hallway smiling.

Me: Wait, what just happened?
Joe: Ashley told us she was taking care of rehab for Mom. Damn, she is your daughter.
Me: What do you think? Mom was a little tough in the hospital, I don't want her to…
Joe: My mom won't…
Me: Of course she wouldn't, intentionally, but if she's frustrated she can become…
Joe: I think we have Ashley do this. It will be good for Mom… and good for Ash.
Me: Okay…wait, what do you mean "She's my daughter"? My goodness, she is doing exactly what you would do, putting her grandmother ahead of anything else and, honestly, she's not thinking through how it will affect her school, her job, and those around her.
Joe: Really? (tension rising in his voice) I don't think of how my actions will affect others?

My head starts to throb, I know that comment was uncalled for. I was reacting to trying to protect my baby from the difficulties that could arise with Mom. I wasn't being fair. Joe always thinks through his actions, he weighs the good, the bad, and the ugly. He makes suggestions and decisions based on how it will help everyone else before himself.

Me: That came out wrong, sorry.

Joe: (shaking his head) She is you, you know.

Me: What does that mean?

Joe: She just told us how we were going to handle the scheduling, no discussion, no consider this or consider that, just, "I will take her and you will work around my class schedule."

Joe sipped his coffee while he intently watched me over the top of his cup.

Me: Well...I...don't...(squirming a little against the kitchen counter). You make it sound like...

Joe: Like you're a little bit of a control freak?

Me: Hey!

Joe: (placing his coffee on the counter and wrapping two very warm, large hands on my cheeks) You are. And while you drive us all a little crazy, we all love you.

Me: (reluctantly accepting the kiss on my forehead) But...

Joe: She's you, Honey (chuckling). I wouldn't dare tell <u>her</u> that, but she is.

I pulled away a bit, not sure about the feelings I was having. I was proud of my baby, but also worried that this new time with her grandmother could change how she saw Mom. She enjoyed a very special relationship, one that started the day Ashley entered the world.

Me: Honey? Promise me we'll ask her every day if it's getting to be too much? I don't want her resenting Mom. She's still young, will she understand if Mo...

Joe: Shhh. Stop, she's so much stronger and capable than you give her credit for.

Me: (sighing) Okay.

I pushed off the counter and headed toward the coffeepot. I had selfishly agreed mostly because I didn't feel I could dedicate more time to the cardiac rehab appointments. I refilled my coffee mug, craned my neck to see the time on the stove, and then looked back at Joe.

Me: I gotta get going.
Joe: Okay (looking down at his feet, while absent-mindedly turning the cup in his hand). I'm right on this.
Me: We'll see.

I climbed the stairs, rolling in my head all the possibilities of what could go wrong with this scenario. Admittedly, I don't like to be proved wrong, but proved wrong was exactly what I was. Ashley and Mom had some of the best days of their relationship during that cardiac rehab. True to my amazing daughter's character, she was Mom's biggest cheerleader. Ashley made exercise fun. She made Mom laugh and become excited about attending rehab. Ashley was known for skipping up the stairs of Fred's house to pick Mom up, singing all the way and totally setting the tone for the day. They would, on occasion, grab a healthy lunch together and spend time just chitchatting. I'll never forget the big deal she made when Mom "graduated." She hung the certificate of completion on the fridge, even celebrated with a visit to Perk on Main, one of Mom's favorite local restaurants, for a heart-healthy lunch, followed up with selfies to share with the family.

Joe shared with me, months later, that he had asked Ashley about taking Mom to rehab the day before the kitchen discussion. They had come to a decision that Ashley would be the primary partner in this little chapter. He is a wise man; he knew I would try to take on the responsibility. He also knew time was taking Mom from our children. This would prove to be a beautiful way for Ashley to spend some very precious time with her grandmother.

As the memory slid away, I refocused on the picture on Facebook. What a beautiful old soul my baby was. I wiped a tear from my cheek. I knew the days of cardiac rehab were challenging to say the least, but Ashley rose to the occasion, never losing her positive attitude, her cheerleader approach. She never forgot the woman her grandmother was, who she was helping, even though she was slipping away right before her eyes. Ashley, at her tender age, already knew we had to cherish every moment we could.

My fingers hovered over the keyboard. How did I tell this wonderful child what a blessing she was? I began to type, then backspaced, then typed again, then backspaced again, deleting my words. It wasn't possible to express everything I needed and wanted to say in such a short blip of a statement.

"I love this post…XOXO…" is what I left in her feed. Of course I made sure I used the ellipses points twice because it drives her crazy when I do!

Ashley had written, "I cherish the privilege of keeping her strong spirit alive." What poignant wise words. I often wonder how my children will keep the memories, the energy, of their grandmother alive, the woman they knew before this illness robbed us of her. I know I will cherish their reflections, after all, they help keep my own crystal clear.

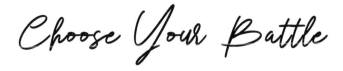

Choose Your Battle

Connecticut

February 2018

I peeked my head into the dining room, which was bustling with activity. Whitney Houston was belting out "I'm Every Woman" from the boom box on the counter, an aide holding a food tray was shaking her hips slightly to the beat and singing along. I smiled and waved to Dorothy, who looked right through me. She was in a special place in her mind, smiling and bouncing her head slightly to the music. I scanned the room for Mom, she was nowhere to be found.

It was exceptionally quiet in the hallway as I made my way through the Star Unit. Josh, an aide and one of the largest, most gentle men I've ever met, approached me with a warm smile. His frame towered over me as I stopped to exchange pleasantries.

Me: Hey! Happy Saturday!
Josh: Hey back at ya! How yous today?
Me: I've got no complaints!
Josh: Gurl, you always say that!
Me: Life is good, my friend, life is good. I'm on the right side of the daisies, what can I complain about?!

Josh threw his head back, letting out a hardy laugh. I basked in the beauty of his energy. His large hand waved me by as he shook his head and smiled at me.

Josh: Ain't that the truth!

Me: Sure is. Hey, Rosemary's not in the dining hall?

Josh: She wasn't having nothin' to do with going to dinner today (shrugging). I tried, but yous know how it is sometimes.

Me: Oh, I get it.

Josh: You choose your battles (chuckling lightly). We'll get her a tray.

Me: Thanks! Catch ya later, friend!

Josh: Yep!

I pushed my hand against Mom's slightly closed door. The room was dimly lit, the only the light was coming through the window from the twilight sky. It was a typical scene of late—a quiet, dimly lit room, the curtain drawn two thirds around her space, and her white Velcro sneakers peeking out from the foot of her bed. I knew when she was having a rough afternoon the best thing for her is quiet space, although it still saddened me that she was all alone in her room. I approached and cautiously pulled the curtain back. There she lay, sound asleep.

Me: (placing my hand on her arm, speaking just above a whisper) Hey there, Beautiful!

MIL: (eyes popping wide open and her arm recoiling from me) Huh?!

Me: Hi, how are you?

MIL: Good? (studying me hard)

Me: Glad to hear it (leaning in to place a kiss on her forehead).

As I pulled back, I saw her face had softened, her eyes were closed, and a tender smile graced her lips.

Me: How about I use my magic wand and sit you up?

MIL: Huh?

Me: Watch this…

I leaned down and picked up the bed control in my left hand, purposely hold-ing it below the bed. As I pretended to wave my "magic wand," I pushed the "up" button for the head of the bed.

Me: Abracadabra!
MIL: (eyes widening in surprise) How…hey…wow.
Me: (smiling and giggling) I have magic powers!
MIL: You do!

Smiling and shaking my head, I placed the control back on the floor next to the bed. Mom stared at me for a moment, then smiled weakly.

Me: So, what's new?
MIL: (shrugging) I don't…I don't know…

I studied her for a moment, trying to judge how she was. I was tired, and my feet were screaming. I had traveled from North Haven to Suffield to Manchester, finally landing here in Wallingford. I had attended two memorial services, conducted a three-hour client meeting in an unheated commercial space, all in stilettos, before I made it to visit Mom. I needed to dig deep for conversation starters, it would have been so much easier if she had been in the dining room. At least there, I could feed off the other residents. The way I was dressed that day, especially in my dress coat with the thick fur collar, always got ooohhs and aaahhs from the ladies, which made for an easy conversation.

Me: So, I saw Scot and Anna today.
MIL: Oh? (not at all registering who her son and daughter-in-law are)
Me: Yeah, they're doing well. Anna's dad passed away this summer and his memorial service was today.
MIL: Uh huh…
Me: You did a great job with your son Scot, Mom.
MIL: Oh?

She still had no idea who or what I was talking about, so I continued more for me than anything else.

Me: You did, he's a wonderful husband and father. I watched him carefully today, he was a pillar of strength for Anna and the kids. It warmed my heart as I watched him hold Sophia's hand during the slide show. Poor Sophia, she's only fourteen, death is so hard to understand at that age. Theo did well, he looked sad, but he did well. Anna's mom looked wonderful. I don't know how she does it, her skin is flawless! Anna's brother gave the eulogy, he just was re-elected to office. He ran for judge, I believe, and her (a yawn creeping into my jaw) other botr Michl ooks grat too.

MIL: Huh?

Me: Sorry (shaking my head), her other brother Michael looks great too.

MIL: Oh.

Me: Dave and Vi were there too.

MIL: Ummm...

Me: You did well there too, Mom. Dave is also a great husband and father. His boys are quite accomplished. Christopher is a wildly talented musician and Timmy can tear up the tennis court with the best! (a yawn creeping in again)

MIL: Uh huh (continuing to stare blankly)

Me: Then there's Cyndi, your daughter. She lives in Arkansas. Life is busy, we don't catch up much. She's a patient, wonderful Mom. Do you remember her son Cody?

Nothing. *Keep talking she hears you, you can do this!*

Me: Yes, Cody, your grandson. You two had a very special relationship.

When Joe's nephew Cody was born, he had a series of challenges, one of which was being born without eyes. Joe's sister Cyndi was and is amazing, as was Mom.

Me: I remember it like it was yesterday when you packed everything you owned to move to Eureka Springs to help Cyndi with Cody. I was jealous and didn't want you to leave!

I looked to the ceiling and yawned again, with this one, Mom catches the yawn.

Me: Last but not least you did well with your son John too. Like with Cyndi, life is busy and we don't talk much, but I hear their oldest son Rory is an EMT. Kinda cool huh?

I think, *Oh my, this is going to be a long visit.* I'm scrambling for what to talk about, and literally rambling. I'm rescued temporarily by the aide bringing in Mom's dinner tray.

Aide: Here ya go, Rosemary.
MIL: Oh! Good! (showing a burst of excitement)
Me: Dinner's looking good, huh?
MIL: (looking at me like I am crazy) Yesssss…
Me: Well, for the most part, you don't like to miss a meal!
MIL: Yeah…
Aide: Rosemary, do you want to sit in a chair or on the end of your bed?

Mom looked up at her, a little confused, but the aide was quick to act.

Aide: Here, I'll set you up on the bed here and she (nodding toward me) can sit in the chair.
MIL: Okay…

The aide got mom settled and I sat back in the chair. I watched Mom eat, redirecting her to her fork and spoon when needed and intercepting the knife more than a few times.

MIL: (sniffing) Humph.
Me: You okay? You need a tissue?
MIL: (sniffling) Yeah.

I stood up to retrieve some toilet paper from her bathroom. As I returned to the bed, I saw her using her blanket to blow her nose.
Me: Oh, Mom (holding the toilet paper out to her), here, I have tissues for you.
MIL: Oh…

She didn't take the tissue, she looked back at her dinner and tried to scoop up the fruit cocktail with her knife. I wonder why the kitchen even sends the knife.

Me: Mom, how about we try this (handing her the spoon).
MIL: Oh, yeah.

She dug around in the fruit cocktail, eventually filling her spoon with fruit. She sat a little straighter for a moment as she chewed then sniffed again, then twice more.

Me: Need this, Mom? (holding the tissue)
MIL: No…I…got my own…

She picked up the blanket again to blow her nose. I decided at that moment to follow Josh's lead on this one and choose my battles. What good would it do if I kept trying to force the tissue on her? What harm is there in her using the blanket as a tissue?

I sat with her for another half hour as she finished her dinner, continuously redirecting her choice of utensils and ignoring her using the blanket as a tissue and napkin.

MIL: Ahhhh (dropping both hands at her side and looking down at her empty plate).
Me: Was that good?
MIL: Sure was, don't you think?
Me: Sure!
Me: Here…I'll move this tray…
MIL: (yawning) Thank you.

I cleared her tray as she turned to lay back against her raised bed. I busied myself for a moment, packing up her laundry to take with me to wash.

Me: (noticing there were no socks in her dirty laundry) What do you do with all your socks? It's like you've got (turning around to look at Mom) a sock thief!

She was sound asleep. I sighed, looking at her blanket balled up at the foot of her bed. I could see beet juice stains from her dinner among other smudges. I decided not to tuck her in. I left the blanket as was. I placed the bag of laundry on the chair and quietly approached her bedside.

Me: Mom (whispering), I'm gonna go.

MIL: Hmmm (not opening her eyes).

Me: (kissing her forehead) I love you.

MIL: (her eyes still closed) I love you, too.

Me: I'll see you tomorrow with Joe (stroking her hair behind her ear).

MIL: Hmmmmm (her eyes closed with a content smile making her way across her lips)

I softly closed the door behind me. Across the hall is the nurses' station, I saw Josh sitting at a computer.

Me: Hey, friend.

Josh: Hey! How we doin' in there?

Me: Sleeping. Can you do me a favor?

Josh: Sure, whadya need?

Me: Mom needs a new blanket. There was some confusion tonight between tissues, napkins, and the blanket.

Josh: (already standing) Sure thing.

Me: It just wasn't worth it.

Josh: (smiling) Choose your battles! Guuurl, go home, you look tired!

Me: A little...thanks so much for the blanket.

Josh: (walking toward a linen closet) I'll take care of it. See ya.

Me: Have a good night.

I punched the code into the keypad to exit the unit. I think, *Battle...* It is such a strong negative word. I don't like negativity and I didn't like to think of myself battling with Mom. It saddened my heart when I thought that way. I passed another nurses' station and made eye contact with one of them. I smiled, and she returned one of her own along with well wishes for a good evening. I reminded myself that good, positive energy and love was what won every time.

Choosing *not* to engage in a battle was actually a positive action, one that made our time together more enjoyable and better for Mom. I signed myself out in the guest book at the main desk and enjoyed a short banter with a few residents and a guest in the lobby. As I turned toward the receptionist to wave goodbye, she stopped me.

Receptionist: You're always so nice and friendly when you're here!

Me: Only way to be, right?

Receptionist: Well, don't stop. I love seeing you come through that door. You lift everyone's spirts.

Me: I won't. Hey, have a great night and stay warm; it's a little raw and chilly.

Receptionist: I will, you too.

The second set of glass doors slid open. The cold air bit at my cheeks. I pulled my collar closer to my cheeks, battling the bitter air. *How am I going to spin this battle into a positive?* I thought. I really don't like the cold. My mind wandered to what my evening held—a quiet evening with Joe, probably curled up on the sofa watching a movie, and, well cuddling somehow seemed cozier when it was cold outside. I smiled, pleased with myself that I'd found another positive, a skill I'd had to hone during this journey with Mom. The resume I had built over the past few years was extensive; this addition was invaluable. I paused for a moment and silently thanked Mom for the great lessons.

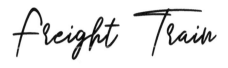

Freight Train

Connecticut

August 2018

I sat in the dealership waiting for a quick repair, I did show up unannounced, so to sit for an hour or so was expected. I busied myself answering a few emails and scrolling through social media. I was trying not to think of everything I could be accomplishing at the studio when a text came in from Joe.

Text from Joe: Mike wants to have dinner tonight.
Text from Me: Okay? Can he come toward us?
Text from Joe: He'd like to show us the house.
Text from Me: Okay.

As I simultaneously scrolled Facebook, I saw someone had liked a recent *Life with MIL* post. I hesitated and scrolled on. My phone signaled another text from Joe.

Text from Joe: We'll leave as soon as I get home.
Text from Me: Okay text/call me when you leave FH.
Text from Joe: K.

Mark from the service department let me know they were almost done with my car and that they were taking it through a quick wash in a minute. I thanked him and told them there was no worry.

Still scrolling Facebook, I saw another "like" pop up from the previous Sunday's post about Snapchat with MIL. I stopped and opened the post, thinking *That's odd...in only a few minutes MIL has popped up in my Facebook feed twice.* I dismissed the tug I felt and chalked it up to coincidence.

Mark: All set, Lis.
Me: Aw, thanks Mark, you're a lifesaver.

I settled my debt and walked to the car. As I placed my hand on the door handle, I felt that tug again. I shook it off and slid into the driver's seat, looking at the clock on the dash, 3:45 p.m. I sighed and thought, *I'll never get anything done if I go to the studio now.* There it was again, a tug. I dialed the studio, deciding to respond to this overwhelming feeling pulling at me.

Sara: Hello?
Me: Hey, I'm gonna stop by and see my mother-in-law unless you have something pressing for me.
Sara: Nah, nothing you can't do in the morning.
Me: Okay, I have dinner plans tonight and I'm feeling like I need to see her.
Sara: Sure, I'll see you in the morning.
Me: Thanks, Sara. Have a great night, sorry you were alone all afternoon!
Sara: Don't worry about it; it was quiet, and I got a lot done!
Me: Thanks. Have a good night.
Sara: You, too.

I glanced down at the gas gauge, a quarter of a tank. The drive out to dinner with Mike would suck that down and more. I turn into the gas station. As the gas pumped, I grabbed my phone and sent Joe a message.

Text from Me: Going to see Mom. It's too late for me to get anything done before we leave for dinner.
Text from Joe: (thumbs up)

I arrived at Regency House and signed in at the front desk while residents gathered, chatting about the weather and Labor Day visitors. I shared some quick greetings and headed down the hall.

Tug...

As I approached the Star Unit, a nurse I haven't met stopped me. Her nametag read "Sue."

Sue: Hi! Who ya heading to see?
Me: Hi! Oh, Rosemary.
Sue: Oh, you must be her daughter-in-law. I see your husband a lot, right?
Me: You probably do.
Sue: I'm Sue, the new nurse manager on this floor, you're the home lady... doing the houses right?
Me: (giggling) Designer, yes. I'm a designer. Is that how he describes me? The Home Lady?
Sue: (laughing and throwing her hand up) Oh, not at all, but it's how I talk to Rosemary about you.

Sue punched in the code to access the unit. I tilted my head and looked at her a little surprised, albeit pleasantly, that the nurses talk about our family, I guess I shouldn't have been.

Me: Really? Thanks...
Sue: Yeah, your husband's the fireman right?
Me: Yep, that's him.
Sue: He's great. We love seeing him (holding the door for me to pass).
Me: (winking) Me too! How's she doing today?
Sue: I'm just coming on shift. I don't know...
Me: Okay, thanks.
Sue: Nice to meet you!
Me: Likewise!

I waved and said some hellos to other residents as I made my way down the hall. I entered Mom's room; the curtain is closed.

Tug...

I approached the curtain and peeked around the corner; Mom was laying on her bed. It was 89°F today and Mom was wearing her winter coat, tears were rolling down her cheeks.

Tug warranted.

Me: Mom?
MIL: (startled, staring at me with wild eyes) What?!?
Me: (swallowing hard) Hey, Beautiful…you okay?
MIL: (shaking her head as her chin starts to quiver) I…I…
Me: (approaching the side of her bed and sitting down) Shhh…sssshhhhh…
    now, Beautiful, it's okay. I'm here. What's goin' on?
MIL: hhmmblds…I sdhdbld…oooohhhh…I…can…sdhhhhaddd…

I stroked her arm and kissed her forehead.

Me: You feeling sad?
MIL: Yea…(sniffling) yes, sad is the word…I…don…I
Me: You don't know why?
MIL: Hhmmm hhmmm yeah…

I hugged her and moved around the bed to tilt the head of her bed up into a sitting position.

MIL: Wha…What…wat ya doin'?
Me: Sitting you up so I can snuggle with you.
MIL: (a smile crept across her face) Snuggle? Ppsshhhh, snuggle…
Me: Yep, snuggle! Sometimes we need snuggles to get our minds back on track.
MIL: Huh?

I adjusted her pillow as she scooched over in the bed. I took up residency at her side and put my arm around her. She looked up at me and smiled.

Me: Now, isn't that better?
MIL: It is…
Me: You feeling a little happier?
MIL: I guess so…

Me: Hmmmmm, ya know what I say? I say our minds are like freight trains.

MIL: Freed…frraadd? What trains?

Me: Freight. Trains.

MIL: Huh?

Me: It's like this. Sometimes something unpleasant comes across our mind, ya know that little thing like realizing you're out of coffee or stubbing your toe. Then, dang it, it makes us sad, or even mad, right?

MIL: Uh huh…

Me: Well, sommmmetimes, that one little thought can take off like a freight train and the next thing you know, your mind is traveling down the sad road at a buck ten plowing down all the happy thoughts, making you about as sad as you can be. It's hard to pull yourself out of that funk.

MIL: Hmmmm…ya think?

Me: I do think. In fact, I absolutely believe it. Ya want to know what I know? I know how I slow down that freight train, you want to know how?

MIL: (shrugging) How…?

Me: Happy thoughts.

MIL: Huh?

Me: You heard me loud and clear. Happy. Thoughts. Want to try it?

MIL: (sulking a little) Okay…

Me: Let's see, oh I know. I know one thing that used to always make you smile and laugh.

MIL: (perking up a bit) Really?

Me: My babies and spaghetti. Oh my goodness, Ma, you loved watching the kids eat spaghetti when they were babies! You'd sit at the table and watch them try to pick up the slippery strands and feed it into their mouths. They'd open their mouths as wide as possible, tongues twisting, turning, and grabbing at the pieces as they slid from their fingertips. Oh, their sauce- covered faces…and how you would laugh if they were lucky enough to capture one and suck hard to pull it in. They'd suck so hard (making a fishy face) that sometimes their eyes would cross!

I looked over at Mom. She was holding her belly, laughing. Apparently, I illustrated my memory of Ashley and spaghetti quite well, because she wasn't only laughing, she was wiping tears of laughter from her cheeks. I continued story telling for a bit until I was certain the freight train of sadness had left the station.

Me: How you feelin?
MIL: You make me happy
Me: I try.
MIL: I'm so happy you're here.
Me: Me too! I had nothing to do today so I said, "How about I stop in and visit Ma?!" I'm so glad I did.
MIL: Me too…
Me: Let's keep that freight train in check.
MIL: What train?
Me: Nothing, Ma. Nothing…

I leaned down and kissed her forehead and imagined the freight train leaving the station…for a little while at least.

The Art of Conversation

Connecticut

September 2018

I stepped out of the car, firmly planting my foot on the pavement. An orange leaf skipped over the toe of my pink suede shoe. The days were getting shorter, the trees were starting to paint the landscape, and we were embarking on a new path with Mom. I looked over the roof of the car to Joe and nodded to him. He knew I was reminding him to grab the laundry bag from the back of the car. As we made our way toward the entrance to Regency House, he slid his hand into mine.

Joe: So whadya think? She up?
Me: I don't know, the last two times I was here after 6:00 p.m., she was sound asleep!
Joe: (looking at his watch) Maybe we're in luck? It's only 5:45 p.m.
Me: That would be nice. I'd like to see her before I leave in the morning.
Joe: If she's not, I'll just come by tomorrow earlier in the day.

I always felt a pang of guilt when I couldn't see Mom before I traveled. Some trips I came back to the same woman I left, other times she'd spiraled again, slipping farther from our grasp. I wished I knew what I was coming home to each time so I could prepare myself, give myself a pep talk, plan out my visit, etc. But the truth was that there was no preparing on this path that had been carved for us.

Joe opened the door to the Star Unit and placed his hand on the small of my back. Nurse Sue rounded the corner, smiling and brushing the corner of her mouth.

Me: Evening, Sue!
Sue: (swallowing hard and dusting her cheek again) Hey there! Just sneaking a snack in while I can!
Joe: (chuckling lightly) Eat when you can!
Sue: That's the truth!
Me: Mom up?
Sue: Yep! (waving as she continues down the hall)

I'm relieved. I looked over my shoulder at Joe and smiled, he returned the smile with a nod toward Mom's room. My steps had a little skip to them as I entered. She was sitting at the foot of her bed, her shoulders slightly slouched, walker firmly placed in front of her. She was just staring, blankly, at the door.

Me: Well hello there, Beautiful!

Nothing. Mom doesn't flinch, she doesn't acknowledge that I've entered the room, there is no response. I stopped and felt Joe right at my back. I took a deep breath and forced a warm smile. After years of practice with her, I've learned how to make my eyes dance and twinkle by channeling the love. I quickly resurrected memories that made me feel loved, simple little memories, such as the way my kids smelled after a bath, or the first time Joe kissed me, or the feeling of walking through my parents' back door, even today, and always feeling safe and loved. Somehow, even though I'm forcing the feeling, it isn't spontaneous after all, the love radiates from me. More often than not, Mom felt it, too.

Me: How you doing tonight?

Mom turned her eyes toward me and I knew immediately she had no idea who was standing in front of her. Was she feeling the love?

Joe: Hi, Mom!
MIL: (squinting) Hi?

Me: Look at you, Beautiful, awake, sitting up, hangin' out. You doing okay
    tonight?
MIL: (studying me closely) Yeah?

I moved closer and kissed her forehead. As I stood up, my mind was scrambling
to come up with topics for conversation tonight. I never realized how difficult
it was to have a one-sided conversation until Mom started to slip away. Those
one-sided conversations were becoming more and more the norm. While she
didn't respond, I still believed she was there somewhere, so I kept trying. I
stepped back, kicked the toe of one pink suede stiletto forward, shifted my
hip, and struck a pose.

Me: Well, Beautiful, whadya think?!
MIL: (looking confused) Huh?
Me: (throwing my head back and rustling my hair a bit) Of *this?*

I waved my hand from my shoulder down across my hip. Joe looked at me,
shook his head, and smiled.

MIL: What?
Me: My dress?! Isn't it pretty? It's so colorful…I love the pen and ink styling of
    the pattern (talking too fast and pointing to the pink, orange, and bright
    green of my dress). Look at all the colors!
MIL: Huh? (curling her lip up and pulling her head back)

I remembered to slow down and speak more clearly. In an effort to be silly and
a little funny, I got a little too excited, and confused Mom. In my head a black
clapper board with its thatched arm snapped together with a loud crack. *Take
Two,* I thought. I tried again, this time with much less drama. I waved my arm
across the dress again, slowly, and let it sit on my extended hip.

Me: (slower) So, what do you think, Mom?
MIL: Of what…
Me: My dress (stepping closer and pointing at the hot pink flower). I love the
    colors.
MIL: It is pretty (reaching up and touching the sleeve)…
Me: (sitting down on the bed next to her) Feels neat, huh?

MIL: Uh huh.

Me: It's made out of scuba fabric!

MIL: Scar...scab...(closing her eyes tight then opening one) scad...huh?

Me: Scuba fabric, they make wet suits out of it.

MIL: Oh.

I knew she didn't understand what scuba fabric was, explaining it would be difficult and she most likely couldn't follow the conversation. I looked up at Joe for some inspiration on a new conversation topic. He's just watching his mom. It was important to keep the conversation going. It was equally as important for us as it was for Mom. Without it, what would our visit have been? Us watching Mom? Mom just staring blankly at us? I was always hopeful these conversations would spark something, and she'd know who we were.

Me: Hey! I know what we didn't tell you about!

MIL: (perking up a bit) What?

Me: The Fair! The Durham Fair was this weekend.

MIL: Oh, was it?

Me: Your son here did an amazing job keeping people safe, finding parking for more than 150,000 people, and so much more.

MIL: Oh?

Me: (wondering if she's really following me) Yep! We had eight inches of rain in one day (leaning down and holding my hand off the floor about eight inches). About that much rain! Ppssshhhh we were sloshing all over the place (looking back up at Mom). Don't you think that's a lot of rain?

MIL: No?

Me: No!? (showing no comprehension of what eight inches of rain means). Trust me, Mom, that's a lot of rain in one day. The fields were swamps.

MIL: Oh.

Me: Let me tell you, I walked *soooo* much. Let's see (looking up at the ceiling, then over to Joe). Let's add up how many miles I walked! (opening my phone, I start calling off numbers) nine plus fifteen and a half, plus eleven and a half or so, actually point nine, but we'll call it a half...how much is that honey?!

Joe: Thirty-six.

Me: Whoa, you hear that Mom? I walked thirty-six miles in three days at the fair!

MIL: Oh

Me: I will say, I look mighty amazing in safety orange. The glow it creates on my face knocks years off me.

Joe laughed and shook his head again.

MIL: Uh huh.

Me: Joe doesn't wear safety orange.

Joe: I do, sometimes.

Me: No, you're in that important *black* polo.

MIL: Oh.

Me: (leaning in close to Mom) I'll admit, he almost looks as handsome as he does in his lieutenant's uniform (opening my eyes wide, smiling, and wiggling my eyebrows for effect).

MIL: Oh.

Me: Yeah, it was quite a fair. I was exhausted afterward. I mean, it's tough work keeping everyone in those bus lines! I had to be creative, you know.

MIL: Huh?

Me: (standing up) Yep! I had to remind people of what it was like to be in grammar school again!

Mom watched me intently.

Me: I'd stand in the line and say, "Okay, everyone, follow me, take one giant step to the right!"

As I said this, I picked up my right leg, bent it at the knee, stretched it out far to my right, and firmly planted it on the floor with a strong stomp. This was not an easy feat in stilettos.

MIL: (a smile creeping across her face) Hmmmm…

Me: (giggling lightly) You would have found it entertaining, Ma.

MIL: Oh.

Me: Yeah, the fair was fun. A lot of work, but fun.

MIL: I didn't go…

Then I felt torn. I was happy Mom was engaging in the conversation, but guilty because she then felt like she had missed out.

Me: Not this year, Mom. It's been a few years since we've taken you. You tend not to be a fan of crowds.

MIL: No...yeah...

Joe: It was crowded this year.

Me: Sure was.

MIL: oh

Me: One of my jobs was taking the honey wagon through the grounds when we had people there.

MIL: Oh.

Me: I'd walk through the crowds yelling at people to step aside...

MIL: Hmmm...

I'd lost her again. I looked up a Joe.

Me: Yeah, you would have found it funny, Mom (giggling a little). I was leading the caravan, Joey and his friend were on quads in front of the honey wagon and I'm complimenting the crowd for listening so well. I said (giggling), "Ya'll listen better than my kids! Thank you!" (starting to laugh a little harder). Then Joey yells out, "Hey I'm your kid!" Oh, Mom the crowd loved it! We really hammed it up (slapping my leg). I mean seriously if you're gonna bring a honey wagon through all those people, ya gotta make it fun right?

MIL: Oh.

I looked over at Joe, it was exhausting carrying on this one-sided conversation. I was quickly running out of things to talk about. I didn't realize how the exchange in a conversation prompts more to talk about. It requires some creativity to carry on by yourself, it's a little like talking to a wall.

Joe: How ya doing, Mom

MIL: (yawning) Hmmm?

Me: Do you want to lay back and get cozy?

MIL: Huh?

Joe: Here (walking around me and raising the head of the bed), we'll get you settled.

MIL: Oh.

Me: (standing up and pulling back the blanket and sheet) Here ya go, Beautiful (patting my hand on the bed).

MIL: Yeah, okay (settling herself into the bed as Joe slid her shoes off her feet).

Joe: I love you, Mom (leaning down and kissing her forehead as I tucked the sheet under her chin).

MIL: (smiling) Hmmmm, love you, too.

Joe: I'll be back tomorrow (kissing her again, this time holding his lips against her forehead for a moment longer). Sleep well

Joe stroked her head for a moment, then looked up at me.

Me: Goodnight, Beautiful, let the sandman come.

I leaned in for my own kiss, as I did she puckered her lips for a kiss back, which made my heart swell.

MIL: Hmmmm.

I stood and turned on my heel and started to leave the room. Just before I reached the door, I hesitated and looked over my shoulder. The sandman had swept her away, a wonderful escape for her. I was determined that next visit I would be even better prepared with more to talk to her about, more memories and more funny stories.

Joe: Hey, its date night (smiling at me). Where ya want to go for dinner?
Me: Yeah! Where you thinking?
Joe: Maybe close to home?
Me: Sounds perfect.

I leaned in and slid my arm around his waist. I wondered what I would return to after my trip. How much more could she slip through our fingers?

Airport Reflection

Florida

July 2019

There I sat, in the Southwest International Airport, three and half hours before my flight because I didn't know what else to do.

I rolled my head forward, lifted my shoulders, and focused on two guests sitting across from me laughing. Two women, one middle-aged and the other elderly. The elderly woman playfully leaned into the middle-aged woman's shoulder and gave her a gentle shove with her own. The middle-aged woman made an over exaggerated expression of astonishment. I watched, trying hard not to be obnoxious. I loved seeing this presentation of a beautiful relationship, one of what mutual love, respect, and friendship looked like, one I knew so well.

My throat began to close, my eyes burned. I blinked three, four times and raised my head to look at the ceiling. I felt my neck, then my cheeks, start to heat up, my eyes darted to the left, then to the right, my chin quivered. *Don't lose it, Lisa,* I shouted silently to myself. I drew a deep breath in through my nose as my chest rose. A single tear escaped my eye and rolled down my cheek. I closed my eyes and leaned my head back, listening to the two women giggle and converse as I reflected on the past five hours.

LISA DAVENPORT

I slid the door to the lanai closed and stopped for a moment to take in my view over the pond. I was basking in the beauty of what lay in front of me, the sun was shining, the water sparkled like little diamonds dancing all along the top. I was smiling, thinking about Joe arriving in a few days. This new life we'd started was filled with challenges, but we were blessed with a strong, stable marriage. My phone began to vibrate on the dining table. I turned and picked it up, studying the caller ID. The only announcement was Wallingford CT. I knew Joe was already home from his overnight shift, the only other option was Regency House.

Me: Hello?
Barbara: Helllow? Lizzza?
Me: Yes, this is Lisa.

I recognize the thick eastern European accent of Barbara, a Star Unit nurse, immediately.

Barbara: Lizzza…ummm this is Barbrah at de Regency Houzzz.
Me: Barbara, is everything okay?
Barbara: Ummm…Lizzzzza, we tried to caul your huzzzband.
Me: It's okay, Barbara, what going on?
Barbara: Rozemarrrry she, she coallapze at breakfast, we call ambulenze…we know there dis…
Me: It's okay, Barbara is she still there, at Regency?
Barbara: Nurse Suppppervizor, here you talk to her.
Me: Yes, please.
Annette: Lisa?
Me: Yes?

My heart was racing.

Annette: I'm sorry, Lisa, we had to call 911. Your mother-in-law lost consciousness during breakfast. She came to with very low blood pressure, and she was complaining of pain in her chest. I was thinking a heart attack, so we called 911, we had to.

256

I am roused from my memory by the sound of the loudspeaker announcing flights. I sipped a very tall cold Mojito and watched the women again. The younger woman adjusted the neckline of the elderly woman's sweater, then gently patted her knee. The elderly woman accepted the help with a weak smile.

Joe: Hello? (sounding distressed and even a little anxious)
Me: Regency House called.
Joe: Yeah, Rick was on shift. (Rick is a medic who works with Joe.) He called, they're enroute to Midstate with Mom. Why didn't Regency call me? (fiddling with his phone) Oh, wait, yes they did. I was vacuuming, I didn't feel my phone vibrate…but Rick called and said they had her and I'm on my way now. What did they say to you?

I gave him the blow by blow of what I knew.

Me: I told them they did the right thing. They seemed so concerned that they called 911. I think because of the DNR?
Joe: Yeah, maybe. I gave Rick a good medical history, I'll probably beat the ambulance to the hospital. I'll update you when I get there. I should probably text my brothers…
Me: I can if you want.
Joe: No, I will.
Me: Wait, don't do it while you're driving.
Joe: I won't. I also want to see what's going on with her.
Me: I'm sorry I'm not there. Should I come home now?
Joe: There's no sense in you coming home 'til we know what's going on.
Me: Okay, keep me posted.
Joe: Yep.
Me: I love you (a tear sliding down my face)
Joe: Love you, too.

I hit "end" and placed the phone on the table. I looked around the condo, less than five minutes ago the energy in this room had been so happy it was almost giddy. Now all the wind had been sucked out of my sails. Waves of guilt washed over me. Currently 1,600 miles sprawled between myself, Joe, and...Mom. In front of me the warm, vibrant sun shone over the glistening pond, songbirds soothed as the fountain splashed, yet I felt black, heavy, ever-so-threatening storm clouds rolling in—it was like the unsettling screech of an angry black crow and that sick feeling that settles into the pit of your stomach when true fear creeps in and takes its awful grip.

The doorbell chime jolted me back to my current reality. I realized I had made plans to spend the afternoon on the beach with my dear friend Shelley. I took a deep breath and walked to the door. Should I cancel? Should I go?

I gripped the door handle with no definitive answer and swung the door open. There stood Shelley, her bright blue eyes dancing, her fresh freckled face breaking into a vibrant smile. I could feel her friendship wash over me.

Shelley: Hey!
Me: Hey...oh, Shelley (the smile falling quickly away from my face).
Shelley: What's up?
Me: Joe's mom has been taken by ambulance to the ER (leading Shelley down the hall).
Shelley: Oh, no...should we reschedule? Do you need to go?
Me: Joe says there's no sense in coming home right now.

I looked up at Shelley, concern filled her face. I knew sitting in the condo by myself would only spin the current pit in my stomach into an ulcer, I needed the distraction.

Me: Really Shell, what can I do? I'm 1,600 miles away. I'm sick I'm not there, but until he says I need to go, really what am I going to do? Sit and hold the phone?

The loudspeaker at the airport signaled another arrival and gate change. The women across from me are still chatting. The middle-aged woman pointed down the hall toward one of the convenience stores. The elderly woman shook her head left to right and waved her hand in a dismissive fashion. As the middle-aged woman stood, she rested a hand on the elderly woman's shoulder and leaned in, speaking in her ear. The woman nodded and patted the middle-aged woman's hand. I watched her walk away; she looked over her shoulder twice in the fifty feet she needed to walk to the convenience store. The elderly woman watched her for a moment, then looked out the window. I watched the middle-aged woman step into the store and take two waters out of the cooler. Before she went to the counter, she walked to the edge of the store and looked down the hall. The elderly woman was now looking around the gate, as if she lost something or someone. The middle-aged woman started to wave. I watched the internal struggle start within her. I can almost hear her thoughts: *Does she see me? Should I go to her now…or can I pay for these waters first?"* The elderly woman saw her, recognized her, and waved. I looked back and forth between the two of them as little waves of relief flew across both their faces.

Shelley climbed onto the tram and adjusted her bag to make room for me in her row.

Shelley: I'm so sorry you and Joe are going through this.
Me: I feel so guilty right now, he's there all alone.
Shelley: I know. It just sucks.
Me: It's not only that. I was home for two weekends. I thought about going to see Mom every day that I was there, but I didn't (swallowing hard). I didn't go, Shelley, because I wasn't in Connecticut that long and honestly, I wanted the time I was

there with Joe to be stress-free. She can no longer really interact with us, she just sleeps or struggles to make sentences. It hurts my heart so much to see her like that. I don't know how to be with her anymore...and it's just so painful to watch Joe look at her. It is just so sad. Now I feel even more horrible. I was never afraid of this dreadful disease...I have faced it head-on like a real trooper, but now...I just feel so awful.

Shelley: Oh, Lisa. You have to know those feelings are under-standable and very real. It's okay.

Me: They may be understandable and real, but it doesn't make them right.

Shelley: She knows you love her; Joe knows you love her. Don't beat yourself up.

I turned my head and wiped a tear.

Me: So sorry to be such a downer today. It's really not like me.

Shelley: If you weren't feeling some of this, I'd be concerned. The break today will be good for you. By the way (pointing out over the inlet as the tram swept by) this is gorgeous!

Me: I know, see why we love it here?

Shelley: Sure do.

The middle-aged woman sat down and handed the elderly woman a water bottle. She watched her struggle a bit to open it, but only for a moment. I guessed she knew the elderly woman wouldn't be able to crack the cap but was acutely aware of walking the fine line between helping and not making the older woman feel like a child. The middle-aged woman seemed to put a little extra struggle into opening the bottle than was necessary. I watched as the elderly woman almost looked relieved that her companion had difficulty, too. When she finally cracked the top, she leaned forward and said something to the elderly woman. I could almost predict what the comment was. Something like, "That stinker was really on tight! I thought I was going to have to enlist the help of that young, strong gentleman over there!"

I watched as the elderly woman smiled and laughed before taking a long swig from the water bottle. I followed the younger woman's hand as she slid it into her jacket pocket. She slowly and slightly dramatically pulled a candy bar from its hiding place. The elderly woman's eyes became wide and excited; her mouth formed a perfect wrinkly "Oh" as her bent finger pointed to her own chest. A smile filled the middle-aged woman's face as the elderly woman took the bar. I felt as if I was trespassing on their private time together, but I couldn't pull my eyes away. I watched closely, wondering if they knew what the future held for them.

Me: Two sand chairs and an umbrella please. Anywhere is fine (turning to Shelley), you okay with that?
Shelley: Yeah...of course!

We followed the path the young man started on his quad. The wind tipped my hat and the salt air changed the texture of my lips. The blue gray sky fell into the blue green Gulf of Mexico with almost no definition. I paused, hesitating for a moment, and watched the water lap up onto the shore. Shelley was laying out her towels and settling in. I was looking for the ocean to wash away the pit that continued to rise in my stomach.

Shelley: (standing and throwing her towel onto the chair) I think I'm going to hop in. Just to cool off a bit.
Me: I'll come for a quick dip, too. I don't want to be without my phone for more than a few minutes.

The water was warm, the sand massaged the soles of my feet. I let the saltwater wash over me. I looked back at our chairs and felt a pull.

Me: Shell, I'm going to go back in...don't rush...
Shelley: I'll come, too.

As I sat in my chair and slid my sunglasses on, my phone chimed. I opened it to Joe's text.

Text from Joe: She's in a lot of pain. Nurse is thinking UTI.
Text from Me: Okay. As we know, those run wild through ALZ patients. I'm surprised she hasn't had more.

There was no answer from Joe as I anxiously waited. Five to seven minutes passed before my phone chimed again.

Text from Joe: She could be bleeding from somewhere, just got the bloodwork back. Hemoglobin's very low.
Text from Me: Oh no…
Text from Joe: We have some decisions to make. I'm good with just making her comfortable.
Text from Me: I agree….I am so sorry I'm not there with you.
Text from Joe: Love you. I'm doing fine.

The elderly woman pulled at the candy wrapper, there was determination laced with frustration on her face. The middle-aged woman patiently watched her. The elderly woman pulled hard and the candy bar jumps free, hopping up above their shoulders, doing its own little acrobatic act. The middle-aged woman didn't miss a beat. In one swift sweep, she caught the bar before it hit the floor. She handed it back to the elderly woman as if catching flying candy bars was an everyday occurrence. I chuckled lightly and silently cheered for this middle-aged woman.

The sun beat down onto the Gulf Shore, although with the breeze it was quite comfortable, almost relaxing. Shelley was doing an amazing job of distracting me with conversation, stories, and just stuff that involved anything except what was happening 1,600 miles away. I was very grateful for her friendship, her

companionship, and I forced myself to focus on what we were talking about. Then my phone rang. The screen announced it was Joe calling.

Me: Shell, this is Joe (throwing my legs over the side of the chair to get up). I gotta take it.
Shelley: Go, take it…go…

I walked toward the berm; the sea grass moved softly in the breeze.

Me: Hello?
Joe: (silence)
Me: Honey? Can you hear me?
Joe: Yeah,…I can hear you…
Me: You okay?
Joe: (drawing in a quick breath) Ummm…(sniffling) ummm…
Me: Oh (my throat tightening), Honey?

I could feel the ball of sorrow as it rose in my throat. I literally ached for him, for Mom, for us.

Joe: Am…am I doing (his voice cracking)…am I doing the right thing? (sniffling). I know we talked…

He fell silent. I imagined him leaning against the wall in the ER, his shoulders slumped, his head hanging, his face red. I bet he was pinching the bridge of his nose and had his eyes squeezed tightly shut. The tears burned and flowed fast as they rushed down my cheeks. How can I be so far away?

Me: Honey?…We…we did talk about this (sniffling). Oh, God, I can't believe I'm not there.
Joe: She's not my mom anymore…she (sniffling). She hasn't been for a very long time.
Me: No, she hasn't been…

I looked up, hoping the salt breeze would dry my tears.

Me: She's been gone for years.

Joe: But, who am I to say if someone (voice cracking again) should live or die?

Me: You're not making that decision. Your mom chose you to be her guardian. She did it…

Joe: She chose me and Scot.

Me: Yes, she did choose you and Scot, but I know why she chose you. She knew you would always be her advocate, you wouldn't waiver, you'd think with a clear mind and you would never not let her wishes be granted.

Joe: It's a lot (blowing out a long breath)…I don't know if I can do it…

Me: (my voice quivering) I know it's a lot, I know you're strong, and I know you aren't selfish. Letting her go is selfless (sniffling). Something I hope and pray you can do for me if it is ever me laying there.

Joe: Don't say that…

Me: But…but that's what love is…

Joe: I know….You're right….I know it's the right thing…it's just so hard…

Me: What can I do?

Joe: Nothing right now (sighing deeply). I've got to call my brothers, this can't be only my choice.

Me: You okay?

Joe: Grrreaaat!

Me: Scot will follow your lead.

Joe: I think so…let me call them…

Me: Call me back, okay?

Joe: Yep…

Me: I love you…

Joe: Love you, too…

I walked back to the chairs where Shelley had just returned from another dip in the gulf.

Me: Hey how about food? Want some lunch?
Shelley: Yea, I'm starving. Joe okay? How's his mom?
Me: Let's order lunch and an adult beverage. I'll update you.

I leaned forward and caught the straw between my lips. The refreshing mojito slid down the back of my throat as I continued to watch my new friends. The elderly woman was fidgeting, folding and unfolding her arms. She opened and closed a magazine, sighing deeply and often. The candy bar was gone, that little reprieve had been short-lived. I watched as the middle-aged woman continued to keep her entertained, never looking annoyed, never losing patience, always kind and loving. Another tear fell into my mojito.

Shelley: If I get fries, will you eat a few?...just a side of fries is what I'm thinking.
Me: Sure, I never say no to fries.
Shelley: So, what are the updates from Joe?
Me: Just that he got them to give her some pain meds and she's resting more comfortably.
Shelley: Are your kids around?
Me: Ashley's working. Remember the pig ate her phone?
Shelley: (swallowing hard after her sip of wine and giggling) Oh yeah! How is she texting you?
Me: Off her computer, I bet she'll call when she's on a break. I want to check in with Joey to see if he can stop in at the ER. I know Joe will say he doesn't need him, I need Joey to do that. Let me call him.
Shelley: I've got a feeling he's on his way already.

Joey: Hello?
Me: Hey, Baby...
Joey: Hey...

Me: I know you're probably at the fairgrounds, it being Sunday and all, but I think I need you to go to the ER and check on Daddy...
Joey: Ma?
Me: Yeah?
Joey: I'm already on my way.
Me: (tears welling up fast) Oh, Baby...I'm so proud of you... thank you...
Joey: I can't leave him there alone.
Me; Okay, let me know how he's doing. Love you.
Joey: Love you, too.

Shelley: He'll go?
Me: He was already on his way.
Shelley: You've got great kids.
Me: Yes, we do.

My phone chimed on the table, indicating an incoming text.

Shelley: Is that Ashley?
Me: No, it's Joe.

Text from Joe: I think you should come home.
Text from Me: I'll find a flight.

I looked up at Shelley. I was scared.

Shelley: What did he say?
Me: I need to go home.
Shelley: Well, let's get you there then.

The middle-aged woman stood with the elderly woman in line at the gate. As they walked behind two other passengers, I watched her gently guide the elderly woman back into line when she started to stray. She handed the elderly woman her ticket, after all they were just steps from the ticket agent.

When they approached the scanner, the woman had nothing in her hand. The middle-aged woman handed both of their tickets to the agent. I suspected she had seen the ticket drop and picked it up for safe keeping. She lovingly rested her hand on the elderly woman's shoulder and helped escort her down the jet bridge. I thought, *What a journey they have ahead of them.* I sent them a silent prayer.

I sat back in my seat and watched the jet bridge door close. As another tear ran down my cheek, I wondered, *Is this the beginning of the end?*

Beginning of the End?

Connecticut

July 2019

The clock read 1:38 a.m. as I leaned across the bed and stroked his forehead.

Joe: (one eye barely open) Hey, Beautiful.
Me: Hey (placing a kiss on his brow).

I watched him for a moment, the splendid escape of sleep had stolen him. It was much needed and well deserved.

Wound a little too tight from too much caffeine, too many hours in an airport, and a long ride from New York, I stretched and willed that same escape to visit me soon.

With freshly brushed teeth and squeaky-clean face, I climbed into bed. With almost twenty-nine years of marriage behind us, our patterns run deep. As I laid down, Joe's arm slid over my waist and pulled me close. My body fit perfectly against his, like a puzzle piece finding just the right place. The rhythm of his breathing returned to a soft snore, which, coupled with the warmth and safety of his body, quickly granted me my own escape.

Not enough hours later, the mattress shifted slightly, gently drawing me from my slumber. I slid my arm across the side of the bed, to find only rumpled sheets. I raised my head, which pounded from lack of sleep, too much caffeine, and most likely not enough water.

Me: What…what are you doing (a yawn escaping) up?
Joe: I can't sleep.
Me: I need fifteen more minutes (throwing my arm over my head).
Joe: (leaning down and stroking the top of my head) You take what you need (gently kissing my forehead). Thank you.

I rolled onto my side, straining to see the clock, 4:53 a.m. My tired, burning eyes shut as Joe closed the bedroom door.

A gentle clink and a warm hand on my cheek awakened me. The mattress sunk slightly at my side as I opened my eyes. Joe holding a cup of coffee was a sight for my tired, sore eyes.

Joe: Good Morning?
Me: (wiping the sleep from my eyes) What time (yawning) is it?
Joe: Just about 7:00. I know it's early, but…
Me: No (pushing myself up on the pillows), I'm getting up.
Joe: Here (handing me the coffee cup).
Me: Oh, you're the best.
Joe: No, you are. What time did you get in?
Me: I don't know, 1:30 a.m.?
Joe: How was the ride?
Me: Not bad after I finally got out of LaGuardia (yawning). That place is a mess.
Joe: Thank you. I know that was a long day.
Me: Thank you? I wish I was here yesterday. Let me get cleaned up and dressed, let's go see her.
Joe: Thanks.

Mom had been released to Regency House after her stay in the ER. Everyone involved thought the familiar surroundings would be to her benefit. While her blood pressure was still low, she was comfortable and relatively alert when she was awake.

I studied Joe and our eyes locked for a moment, then his dropped to his coffee mug. His face told the story of the weight he'd carried for the past eight years thanks to this disease. I reached out and gently squeezed his thigh. He returned the gesture with a weak smile and his own loving caress on my leg.

The ride to Regency House was filled with matter-of-fact conversation. Joe once again was employing that great coping mechanism where he becomes clinical and removes personal element from his situation. He updated me in greater detail on the turn of events from the previous day and the conversations he'd had with the doctors. Once again Megan, the nurse supervisor who had helped us get Rosemary into Regency in the first place, was at the helm helping with details, checking on Mom's plan of care.

Joe: It was great to talk to Megan again.

Me: How is she?!

Joe: She's good. She said that even though she isn't really involved in Mom's care anymore, she couldn't forget her RoRo and wanted to help.

Me: Mom wasn't crazy about that RoRo name early on, but Megan seems to have a way with her; it's nice to know she's watching out for us.

Joe: Yeah, it is. I think Regency was a good choice. Mom even ate dinner last night (shaking his head and slight smile crossing his face), she's a fighter.

Me: How's she doing with just those top teeth?

Joe: Soft foods are working.

I thought, *In the last few months, we've lost her glasses and bottom teeth.* The glasses I understood, another resident could have swiped them, unlikely since they hadn't turned up. She probably tossed them in the trash. I wondered, *Did she toss the bottom teeth too?* I thought, *How she's chewing?* Is it painful with her upper teeth against just her bottom gums? Are the gums so calloused that she doesn't feel it? As these questions and scenarios rolled around in my head I was suddenly brought back to the present moment. A set of very familiar chords fill the car speakers and I quickly look out the passenger side window. Tears sting my eyes as Brad Paisley began to tell the beautiful story I knew so well.

> *When I get where I'm going*
> *On the far side of the sky*
> *The first thing that I'm gonna do*
> *Is spread my wings and fly*

His voice seeped through the speakers; I closed my eyes as a whimper slipped from my lips. The tears flowed as I softly sang the words.

> *Yeah when I get where I'm going*
> *There'll be only happy tears*
> *I will shed the sins and struggles*
> *I have carried all these years*
> *And I'll leave my heart wide open*
> *I will love and have no fear*
> *Yeah when I get where I'm going*
> *Don't cry for me down here*

Me: Honey?

Joe: Hmmmm?

Me: (wiping another tear) This song (pointing to the car stereo)…when the time comes…we have to have this at her (my voice cracking)…listen to the words.

> *So much pain and so much darkness*
> *In this world we stumble through*
> *All these questions I can't answer*

Me: When (gasping)…when she goes, she won't…

Tears streamed down my cheeks as I fought to contain the sobs and collect my thoughts.

Joe: You're right, it's…

> *Yeah when I get where I'm going*
> *There'll be only happy tears*
> *I will love and have no fear*

Me: No fear…no more pain and darkness (sniffling)…she'll have no fear… shit!…I can't stop…can't stop crying…I'm a mess. How am I going to go in and see her?!

I thought about God and his timing as the last chords of Brad Paisley's song faded from the speakers. Joe slid the car into park in the Regency House parking lot. I put my head against the headrest and blew out a long breath, wiping the hot tears from my cheeks. My phone chimed. I flipped it over, fumbling a little trying to focus on the screen. It was a text from Andrew, saying he and Ashley were on their way.

Joe: Who's that?
Me: Andrew.
Joe: Andrew?
Me: Probably Ashley through Andrew's phone. Remember, the pig ate her phone.
Joe: (lightly laughing) Only our Ashley…

Suddenly the thought of the pig eating Ashley's phone struck me as funny. I started to laugh a good hearty belly laugh. The flip of the switch from heartache to amusement reminded me of the hormone rollercoaster I experienced when I was pregnant. Emotions are strange. I was acutely aware I needed to get mine back in check before I entered Mom's room.

Doris sat in her wheelchair by the nurses' station, she turned to see Joe and me entering the unit and started shuffling her chair in our direction. Her round face became animated with the excitement of our arrival. I was instantly torn. While I always felt Doris was starved for attention and deserved a little of my time, my priority right now was to see Mom.

Doris: Hubba…dobab (waving her hand toward us).

Taking a deep breath, Joe passed me and approached the nurses' station. I knew if I was patient with Doris, she'd slow down a bit and I might be able to understand her.

Me: Good morning, Doris (gently stroking her hand).
Doris: (smiling widely) Gould mawwwwing...
Me: How are you today, my beautiful friend? I love your hat!
Doris: (touching the brim of her hat) Ohhhh...a...dabba.

Doris raised her hand, pointing from her head to me. Her eyes became large, wide, round circles as her lips jumped into a rhythm, stretching tightly across her open mouth and relaxing again. She always began this little routine right before she had something important to share. I dug deep for a few more minutes of patience, reminding myself another minute or two with Doris would bring her great joy. I squatted down in front of her chair and stroked her hand.

Me: Tell me, Doris.
Doris: (looking up to the ceiling, then back at me) Dabba...dapp...aye dappiss
Me: (searching her face) One more time, Beautiful, slowly...
Doris: (her mouth flexing and working hard to form the words) Aye...dappiss
    on da offar...may (pointing at her chest)...a dappiss on da offar (her fingers
    dancing in the air).
Me: You were a typist?
Doris: Yo! (smiling).
Me: Doris, I bet you were an awesome secretary...I can just feel it.
Doris: dappiss...yo dappis on offar (smiling and pointing to her chest).
Me: That's great! I'm going to go see Mom now...I'll stop by on my way out,
    okay?

I stroked Doris's cheek for a moment, she leaned her face into my hand as I stood.

Me: See you in a little bit.
Doris: Bub bye.

I stepped through the door of Mom's room; the curtain was pulled, only allowing the view of her feet at the end of her bed. I approached the bed to find Joe sitting at her side holding her hand. She was sound asleep, her mouth wide open. I heard her softly snoring.

It started at my diaphragm and quickly worked its way over my chest and into my throat, the anxiety of the last twenty-four hours escaped and replaced itself with relief mixed with a bit of that regret with which I'd been struggling.

I dropped my purse on the bed table and sat on the very edge of her bed, she barely stirred. I watched her carefully for a moment before I leaned in and kissed her forehead. A tear dropped from my eyes, landing on her cheek. She stirred and struggled to open one eye.

I leaned in close and whispered in her ear.

Me: Thank you. Thank you for being here. I love you so much.

I let my lips sit on her forehead for a moment, as another tear slipped over my cheek and onto her brow. I pulled back and tenderly wiped the tear from her temple before it escaped into her ear.

Me: I bet you didn't expect a shower from me this morning, did ya?

I knew she heard me because she tried to open her eye again, but sleep was the champion.

We sat in silence for close to an hour. Joe brought his mother's hand to his cheek, closing his eyes and bowing his head. His shoulders began to shake as he moved her hand to his lips. I watched, a mix of emotions flowed over me— overwhelming love, loss, grief, gratitude, even a touch of anger. This disease had stolen so much from us. I missed the woman Mom had been, I missed our chats and our time together. However, I am grateful she loved me enough to allow me to be such an intimate part of her journey. I am even more grateful that Joe never pushed me away. I am keenly aware that another man could have handled things very differently.

Joe looked up at me, he looked so tired.

Me: How about some breakfast?
Joe: Yeah, I need to go to town hall for some paperwork.
Me: Ashley and Andrew are still an hour away.

Joe: We need to stop home and pick up her clothes, too…I put them in the dryer this morning before we left.

We gave Mom a little more love before we left. She stirred a bit, but returned to a soft snore quickly.

Breakfast in a classic diner is a comfort meal. I love a diner that catapults me back to *Mel's Diner*. I often secretly look for the local Flo and hope she's our waitress. There's something about the steaming cup of coffee in the classic white diner mugs, the bustle of the short-order cooks, and two eggs over easy with crispy bacon and toast. It is a constant in life, it is expected…it is predictable and certain. With the future so unclear, it was exactly what we needed.

I took a long sip of coffee and watched Joe over my coffee cup. He looked up from his plate as his fork stopped midway to his mouth.

Joe: What?
Me: (lowering my coffee mug) Nothing.
Joe: Nothing?
Me: I was just thinking about how long we've been at this.
Joe: What, Mom?
Me: Yeah…it's gotta be almost eight years?
Joe: (hesitating and looking off over my shoulder for a moment before his eyes return to me) Yeah, I think so…I'm trying to remember. Didn't we start to wonder if she was okay when she forgot to pick Ashley up one day from school?
Me: But Ashley was at Strong that day, Ash graduated from high school nine years ago…I think we realized that during the Yale study…
Joe: When did we start that Yale study?
Me: July 2012? …
Joe: Wow.

I pushed back my now empty plate and caressed my coffee mug. The liquid reflected the recessed can over my head. I became mesmerized by the pattern as I gently spun the mug. My mind wandered through the years we had cared for Mom, not only during this Alzheimer's run but her brush with fasciitis.

Joe: You ready?

Me: (slightly startled, not realizing I wasn't even present) Oh, yep (stealing one last gulp of coffee).

Joe: Is Ashley close?

Me: Yep. Let's grab Mom's clothes and go back. They'll beat us, but maybe a little time alone with her would be good for Ashley.

As we approached the door, Joe placed his hand on the small of my back and guided me through the diner door. I flashed back to walking through this door a year ago when we brought Mom for lunch here. I fought back a tear, realizing that was not in our future anymore.

Her Kindred Spirit

Connecticut

July 2019

I'd recognize those feet anywhere. Peeking out from the room curtain, a pair of Birkenstocks rest on the foot of Mom's bed. A welcome rush of love and joy filled my heart, I will never grow tired of that feeling. My children always bring my world into alignment. As I pulled the curtain back, Ashley's crystal blue eyes rose to meet mine. I was worried that her seeing her grandmother like this would be a lot for her to handle. She either was the master of hiding feelings or, as I would learn in the weeks to come, she was stronger than I ever imagined. Across the bed Andrew leaned against the window, legs crossed at the ankles and his arms casually folded, seemingly comfortable and at ease. I studied him for a moment, looked down at Mom and back at my future son-in-law. There was so much future ahead of us, I hoped I could remember the acceptance and love that Mom showed me. She always treated me as her own child, not just the person who happened to marry her baby. Andrew pushed himself off the windowsill and crossed the room with his arms open, ready to receive me. I allowed his strong embrace to not only offer me comfort, but to solidify a secret promise to follow the example Mom had taught me over the last twenty-nine years, to always love him as my own.

Ashley: Mama, I've been reading recipes to Grandma.

My arms embraced her, I buried my nose in her hair and kissed her head. She looked up with a smile that quickly turned into a crinkled nose as she gently batted away the kisses I continued to cast over her forehead and cheeks.

Ashley: Ma! Okay…It's good to see you, too.

Joe: Thanks for coming, Ash (turning to Andrew and accepting his hug with a strong pat on his back). What is this I hear about a pig and your phone?

MIL: (suddenly raising her head off the pillow) Pag?…Huh? (her eyes cracking open as she attempts to focus on us in the room)…wat?…hhhhmmmm?

Joe: Well, hello there!

MIL: Hello?

A smile crept across my face. I watched as Joe's face relaxed, and he stroked Mom's hand.

Joe: How you doing?

MIL: (yawning) Humph…humpohly…

Joe: That good, huh?

MIL: Yeah…

Joe: Did you see Ashley and Andrew are here?

MIL: Oh? (squinting and looking around the room).

Ashley: Hey, Grandma!

Andrew: Hi there.

MIL: Hi…

Joe: Lisa's here (waving me closer to the bed).

Ashley dropped her feet off the end of the bed, inviting me closer to Mom's bedside. I pushed my handbag farther over my shoulder and leaned down to kiss Mom's cheek. I squeezed onto the bed.

Me: Hey there, Beautiful…Pea 2 here…

MIL: Hmmm…hi…(smiling)

The tears stung as I tried to focus on her face. My hand slid into hers and she gently squeezed it in response. There was energy in that soft grasp that brought me a sliver of peace.

I turned back to Ashley, being conscious of not overstepping her visit with Grandma.

Me: Baby? You want to sit here?
Ashley: Nah, we've been here for a while, you sit.
Me: Thanks. She was asleep when I got here this morning.

I started my typical chatter about the morning ride to the town hall with Joe, those one-sided conversations at which I never excelled. I looked up at Joe and shrugged, wondering if Mom could even hear me.

MIL: Yawwwwn…(her eyes popping wide open) Wellll…Hello there…

A giggle escaped my throat as I watched her literally bounce to life before my eyes. Her eyes were bright. Yesterday I was scared to the core of my being that she was dying and I was 1,600 miles away.

Me: Well…welcome back!
MIL: Yeah?
Me: How you feeling?
MIL: Good…you?
Me: Oh, Mom (shaking my head and smiling). You always keep me guessing.
MIL: Oh yeah?…Good.
Me: Good?

I looked to the other side of the bed, where Joe had settled in.

Me: You hearing this, Honey? She likes to keep us guessing.
Joe: You, maybe. Me? She wouldn't do that to me. I'm her favorite son!
MIL: Yep!
Me: Hey!!!!!

Mom gently laughed as an aide entered the room with her lunch tray.

Me: Lunch? You hungry, Mom?
MIL: Oh, yes (pushing to sit herself up).
Joe: Here, let me sit you up.

281

Joe pointed to my side of the bed. I looked back at him, questioning in my mind what I was seeing. Was it a miracle before my eyes? I was confused the previous day, I thought we were losing her forever. I had been regretting my most recent actions, that morning she had been out cold and pretty much unresponsive to my voice and touch. Just then, she seemed fine, like she did the few weeks previous when I left her.

Me: Okay, Beautiful, let me get my magic wand and abracadabra, I'll raise you up!

As I held the bed control just below the mattress with my left hand, I raised my right hand over Mom's chest. As the head of the bed started to move, I started to close my fingers against my thumb, breaking my wrist into a motion that appeared to be me pulling a string to boost her into a sitting position. I watched her face. There was a time she would have smiled and looked surprised, as if I did have some magical powers. Those days are long gone. Instead of longing for that reaction back, I found myself thankful that she was even responding and looking for her lunch.

Me: There ya be, Beautiful.
Joe: Can you raise the bed so we can slide the tray under it?
Me: Ready? (looking at Mom) Ride two coming up!

I noticed she was studying my face; her eyes were radiating something I hadn't seen in over a year. Joe slid the tray over the bed and started to set up lunch for her. I looked at the tray and wondered how she'd navigate some of the dishes laid out, the egg salad sandwich would be soft enough, and the ambrosia salad should go down okay, but the beet salad…there was celery. I reached over and started to pull the beet salad back.

MIL: Hey (looking at me sharply). What?!
Me: Maybe we should try something else that…
Joe: (recognizing what is starting) That might be a little hard to chew, Mom.

Mom glared at me. I wondered if she could even see me clearly. Her glasses had been gone for months.

Ashley: It's okay, Grandma. Daddy's got other yummy stuff here.
Joe: Here, Mom, how about a sandwich…

Joe started to bring the sandwich to her lips. She grabbed it and took a bite. She raised the sandwich and pulled her arm back as if to throw it at me. I made a face as if I was startled. I forced a smile, hoping my playful approach could defuse this.

Joe: Easy does it, Mom (scooping a helping of ambrosia). Here, this is good.

Mom opened her mouth wide and welcomed the spoonful. As she chewed, a look of satisfaction and grunts of delight filled the room. As quickly as those came, they left as she pushed her tongue out, grabbing remnants of coconut and spitting.

Joe: (grabbing a napkin) Here let me get that (wiping her mouth and chin that are now a mess).
MIL: Yuck (spitting).
Me: Let me get a towel, that way we can put it around her neck, like a bib.

When I returned to the room, I found Ashley, Andrew, and Joe laughing and making conversation with Mom about her lunch. I felt a sense of relief that it now appeared we'd dodged that bullet—the one that arrives with no warning and rips my heart out. The bullet filled with her resentment of me and laced with her belief that I am some kind of threat, all permeated with distaste and hate.

Me: Hey, Mom. I've got this (holding up the towel). Let me tuck this around you…

She looked at me, that gentle smile fell from her face. I watched as her eyes squinted tightly and her lip turned up. I regrettably leaned in and started to tuck the towel around her neck and shoulders. She turned her head abruptly away from me. I looked at Joe, he motioned me away from the bed with a quick shake of his head.

Joe: Let's try some juice (raising the glass to her mouth).

Ashley: (clearly seeing and feeling the tension) I love apple juice, but not with tacos, right Daddy?!

Joe: Oh, yeah, apple juice and tacos are a deadly combo!

Joe and Ashley reminisced about the time I made tacos for dinner. We were out of milk, so I poured four glasses of apple juice. Even as an adult, Joe used to down three to four glasses of milk with his dinner. I used to love watching Joey try to keep up with him. Well, on this dreadful night, Joe still polished off four glasses of apple juice with his tacos. The combination had him in the bathroom before dinner was done.

Ashley: (holding her belly as she laughed) Oh, Grandma, that story *still* makes me laugh!

Joe: And it makes me...well let's just say I *don't* like remembering how I unloaded the apple juice and tacos!!!

As laughter filled the room, I thought I was in the clear and spoke up.

Me: Good thing we're having egg salad for lunch huh Mom?

Mom, holding the sandwich again, raised it and pulled her hand back ready to throw it.

Joe: (intercepting the sandwich) Now, now, how about the beet salad?

I leaned my back against the tall cabinet in the corner and watched Mom forget I was in the room. I was tired, my heart was hurting, I was even experiencing a bit of jealousy that Joe, Ashley, and Andrew could have this visit and I couldn't. I certainly wasn't proud of my resentful feelings, and I knew I needed to stifle them. I pulled my phone from my back pocket, looking for a distraction.

Joe: Wow! You did good!

MIL: Hmmmm yeah, it...(yawning) was good!

Joe: You getting tired, Mom?

MIL: I think so...yeah.

Ashley: Let's get you comfortable.

I watched, remembering getting Mom cozy on our sofa when Fred was at the firehouse or any other evening when we had her for a few hours. Ashley tucked Mom in while Andrew said his goodbye. My daughter's love and compassion poured over Mom. Watching Ashley standing over Mom, I saw again that they were kindred souls, Ashley had somehow absorbed all the wonderful traits I so respected in Mom—empathy, patience, humor, and, her best attribute, the ability to be nonjudgmental.

With caution I approached Mom's bed. As I stroked her forehead, she looked up to me. Our eyes connected and, to my relief, gone was the woman who was ready to throw a sandwich at me.

Me: Hey, Beautiful. We're going to take Ashley and Andrew for some lunch.
MIL: (sleepily) Okay.
Me: I'll see you soon.

I let my lips sit on her forehead for a moment.

MIL: Hmmmm…

Joe gently placed his hand on my shoulder, guiding me out of the room. The warmth, weight, and strength of his hand instilled a sense of comfort and peace in me.

Over a lunch of comfort food—potato skins, wings, sliders, and beer—Joe continued to explain more of what the upcoming weeks could bring. How Mom's medical team was cutting back on her medications, and while comfort measures had been in her file for months now, the staff understood that there would be no more trips to the emergency room. Nature would take its course. This, understandably, raised a series of questions—how long did we have? Would we know when it was close? I watched Joe's face closely as he spoke, he seemed comfortable in talking about the future. He explained that the end could be a week from now or a few months. Mom, despite her health challenges, would constantly keep us guessing.

Me: Do you think…should we cancel your trip to Florida for Valerie's House?
Joe: I think it'll be okay. I think I can go and get back.

Me: What…what if she…

Joe: If Mom could understand what we were doing at Valerie's House, she'd insist we go.

I studied his face. I looked across the table at Ashley and Andrew, looking for validation, but none of us held a crystal ball. I turned from their faces as tears welled up in my eyes again. I watched the bustle of Main Street when a sudden feeling of peace fell like a veil over me.

Me: The sun and salt could be a good break for you, and you're right, she would tell you to go.

Joe squeezed the top of my knee and gave me a weak smile. I looked across to Ashley. Her strength amazed me. Little did I know how strong she would need to be in the very near future.

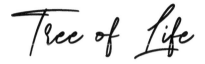

Tree of Life

Florida

August 2019

The tropical air kissed our cheeks as the airport doors opened. Joe slid his hand into mine, preparing to guide me across the road to the shuttle stop. He adjusted his backpack before he stepped to the edge of the curb, looked down at me, and smiled. I reached over and stroked the back of the worn brown leather backpack. Mom gave him that backpack when he entered paramedic school. It had seen years of classes, vacations, hospital stays—both for himself and for Mom. I wondered if Mom knew how special that backpack would become when she gave it to him eighteen years ago. The life it had lived could fill a book.

Joe: Come on (tugging my hand gently), it's clear and I see the bus.

I fell in step, glancing up quickly. His face looked relaxed, something I hadn't seen in months. Maybe he was right, this trip was needed. As we settled into the bus, I exchanged a series of text messages with Katie and Laurie, confirming the delivery of Joe's tree crate.

Me: Crate arrived at the warehouse.
Joe: Awesome…I hope this tree idea of yours works.
Me: I have no doubt.
Joe: I've been going over how to construct it. I think I've got it, but…

LISA DAVENPORT

Me: (squeezing his knee gently) Like I said, I have no doubt.
Joe: It's such a special tree, it's really a cool idea. I think the kids will love it;
Angela will love it.

When we opened LDD Interiors in 2012, both Joe and I felt strongly that we should give back to our communities. In 2016, when we expanded to Naples, Joe met Angela, the founder of Valerie's House, a very special grief center for children who have lost their parents or siblings. Angela lost her mom at the age of ten. For the past three and half years we'd donated our time and resources to Valerie's House's mission. In 2019, Angela secured a rental property for the Naples location, allowing the kids to have a more permanent home instead of meeting in a church hall. Over cocktails and lunch on a sweltering hot May afternoon, I shared with Angela my vision for transforming the rental property from a cold commercial space to a home by using the talents of interior designers across the area. Somehow, we pulled it off. Every room was designed by a local designer who had their designs executed in a mere six weeks. We were now two weeks before the opening, and our space, the gathering room, was still missing its focal point, the tree.

Joe: (unlocking the car door) I think Mom knows we have important work to do.
Me: (looking over the roof of the car) You think so?
Joe: Yeah, I do...I feel...oddly at...peace.
Me: That makes me feel better. I'm so worried she...
Joe: She won't. She'll be there when I get back, I'm only gone four days.

Joe had constructed the base or, better said, tree trunk of our vision in our carriage house in Connecticut. The idea I had was to sculpt a tree out of pieces of old wooden pallets, giving new life to discarded palettes. Now, at Valerie's House, Joe added the limbs. The tree grew before my eyes in the corner of the gathering room as Joe guided the branches to reach and stretch out of the trunk and spread across the walls, over the windows, and onto the ceiling of the room.

We added twinkle lights to give the tree further depth while allowing it to glow with life. I had requested two hundred wooden leaves from Real Wood Floors, a hardwood flooring company with their own mission to help children, and

288

they happily agreed. I had painted the leaves six different happy, bright colors. The leaves were inspired by the children's book *The Fall of Freddie the Leaf* by Leo Buscaglia, which was a book about the circle of life.

As I twisted the cup hooks into the tree branches, I thought of the children who would fill this tree in memory of their loved ones. It would become a tree filled with colorful leaves and children's handwriting. As the kids gathered each week under the tree to share in a meal, above them and around them the twinkling lights would be their special people.

I stepped off the ladder and backed across the room, admiring our work. Joe slid his arm around my waist.

Joe: It's beautiful.
Me: I never doubted it
Joe: Mom would love this.
Me: Yeah, she would.

The next time Joe saw the tree, he'd be asked to honor his own mother. Losing a parent is devastating at any age.

Bathroom Call!

August 2019

I kissed Mom on the head and tucked her in.

Me: I love you, Mom.
MIL: (garbled mumbling) Lum fumb.

I stroked her forehead for a moment and watched a smile creep across her face. The peacefulness radiated from her face as she slowly closed her eyes.

Me: Does that feel good, Mom?
MIL: Hmmmm…
Me: (softly chuckling) How 'bout if I do it until you drift off to sleep?
MIL: (groggily) Hmmm…

The sandman himself quickly swept in and brought Mom to the escape of dreamland. I brushed my lips over her forehead, kissing her goodbye. Quietly, I stood and crept away from her bed to leave her room. I pulled her curtain for privacy and was greeted by Shirley, another resident at her door.

Me: (whispering) Hey there, Beautiful! Can I help you?

She was determined to get into Mom's room and was pushing past me in her wheelchair.

Shirley: I...I...I need to use the bathroom!

Hunched over, slouched in her wheelchair, she continued to shuffle her feet pulling herself farther into the room. She was a woman with a mission!

Me: Well, now, let's see if we can't get you to a bathroom then, okay?
Shirley: (craning her neck to see me better) Yes this is...I need to use the bathroom...

I gently guided her chair out of the room toward the desk, where an aide was reviewing paperwork.

Me: I think Shirley needs to use the bathroom. Do you think you can help her with that?
Aide: Well, Girrrrl! You're the next contestant up! How about that now?!

I giggled and playfully tapped my hip on Shirley's arm.

Me: There you go, Shirley!

I looked over my shoulder back toward Mom's room where her roommate, Christine, was waving goodbye.

Christine: Good nighhhhhtt (smiling and making eye contact).

Her response surprised me. So often she just slept or laid in bed, staring off into space. Not tonight, tonight she was having a good night. I smiled and stopped to chat for a moment.

As I left Christine, I stopped in the hallway and placed myself squarely in front of four ladies lined up in chairs along the hallway wall.

Me: Well, it's that time, ladies! Goodnight! I'll see you soon!

The chatter began, goodnights coming out in all different ways, some fragmented, some clear some just "ya, ya, ya."

I smiled and stepped aside to see the resident marine. I felt a pang of guilt as I smiled at him. Just the other day he had insisted I come sit on his lap during group exercise. Well, in an effort not to disrupt the class, I smiled and shook my head no, which sent him into a full-blown tizzy, disrupting the class anyway! I was thankful that it appeared he'd forgotten my denying his offer to sit on his lap!

Me: Goodnight, kind sir! (bending down so my face was level with his).
Marine: Dhubded (smiling).
Me: You too, Sir. You have a great night!

I waved and started down the hall to leave. I stopped for a moment to say hello to a young girl visiting a resident. As I was about to compliment her on her fun toe polish, I felt a gentle bump on my purse. I turned to see Shirley looking up at me.

Me: Hey ya, Shirley! What's going on?
Shirley: I...I...humph...I...desssprately need to use ummm desssprately need to use the bbb...bathroom.
Me: Okay, we'll get you some hel...
Aide: Girrrlll, where ya goin'? (looking at me and shaking her head)
Shirley: b...bbb . . BATHROOM! I desssprately need to use the bbb... BATHROOM!

Clearly Shirley was getting upset about the bathroom. I touched her shoulder and gave her a reassuring squeeze.

Aide: (ever so gently) I know, Honey. I was getting your shower stuff together! Let's go...
Shirley: bb...bbb...BATHROOM!
Aide: Uh huh...

And then it started, a chorus of requests for the bathroom began—the four ladies, the marine, another voice from another room—all at once they all needed to use the bathroom. A smile turned up the corner of my mouth as I made eye contact with the aide.

Me: Hey, looks like you're in high demand tonight (stifling a laugh).
Aide: (laughing and shaking her head) Gotta love 'em!
Me: Rock on all!

I waved my hand and approached the door to leave. As I closed the door behind me, I saw the marine waving to me; I blew him a kiss. This journey we're on does have silver linings. The patience I've learned with Mom over the years spills into relationships with complete strangers. Many need, and deserve, just a little extra love—spending an extra moment to say goodnight, or finding an aide for a bathroom, an occasional smile and a blown kiss—life is short, love like crazy!

Goodbye, Sweet Christine

Connecticut

August 2019

I glanced down at my watch, 9:30 p.m. A yawn crept up the back of my throat as my bottom jaw fought to keep it from escaping. The tears welled as I lost the battle.

I looked across the bed at Joe stroking Mom's arm, gently "shhing" her between her winces of pain and soft groans. Likewise, I repeated the gentle caress along the length of her very cool thumb. Behind me, Mom's roommate Christine's breaths were raspy, almost rattling, she had been sleeping for days.

Me: Do you hear Christine?
Joe: Hmmm?
Me: Christine, can you hear her breathing?
Joe: (hesitating to listen) Oh…yeah…
Me: That doesn't sound good.
Joe: (shaking his head lightly, the corner of his mouth turning into a frown) It's not.
Me: (swallowing hard) Is that what they refer to as the death rattle?

He didn't respond. He lowered his head and looked at Mom. I looked over my shoulder, craning my neck to try to watch Christine. I saw her Tuesday night when I stopped in to feed Mom her dinner. She was laying peacefully in her bed, she seemed to be beginning to drift off to sleep, the tame flutter of her eyelashes the only motion I could see. I had stopped by her bed to carefully give her warm hand a light squeeze and say a quick hello. She had barely responded. Now, on this late Sunday night, I watched an aide stop by her bed to swab her mouth.

I returned my attention to Mom, the morphine, or "magic juice" as I'd coined it, seemed to have taken her pain. Joe was watching her closely as a yawn escaped him as well.

Me: How ya doing?
Joe: Okay, I think we can head out soon. She seems more comfortable now.
Me: When you're ready.

We sat for a bit longer until the exchange of yawns between us became our queue that it was time for our own rest.

Joe: I think she's okay, let's head out.

I nodded and stood, leaning in to kiss Mom's forehead.

Me: Hey, Pea 1, Pea 2 here. Don't give Yolanda a hard time tonight (kissing her forehead). I love you.

I stepped back and let Joe come around to my side of the bed. He adjusted Mom's blanket, tucking her arms under the soft fabric. He leaned in and kissed her brow, whispering his love.

Joe shut down the light over Mom's bed. I turned to head toward the door. I hesitated at Christine's bed for a split second, her breathing was still the same. I looked down, not liking the feeling that was creeping over me. Joe slid his hand in mine as we walked through the room's door. The hallway was quiet, something I rarely had heard in this unit, the sweet escape of slumber had taken hold of the residents, an escape I couldn't wait to find myself.

The following morning, the sun was bright at our backs as the doors to Regency House slid open. We stepped up to the receptionist's desk and exchanged pleasantries with her as Joe picked up the pen and signed us into the guest book. I looked up at the clock, 8:15 a.m.

The hallways were filled with a bustle, quite the contrast to what we left behind less than twelve hours ago.

Behind the door of the Star Unit, Kathy, one of the residents, was standing at the window looking out. Joe punched the code into the wall pad, unlocking the doors with a soft click. He gently pushed the door open, but only partially.

Joe: Well, good morning!

I squeezed in between the doors and pushed the door closed. Kathy was looking intensely at me. Doris, I discovered, is the reason we can't open the door more than eighteen inches, her wheelchair is almost against the door.

Me: Good morning, ladies! We're up early!
Doris: Dat wought (pointing to the door). Gow outaaa!
Me: Not now, Doris. Breakfast is coming soon.

I looked for Joe, but he was already around the corner and in Mom's room.

Doris: Noooo, gow outtttt (pointing at the door, upset and determined).

I recognized her frustration and decided to defuse it quickly. A soft touch always worked well with Doris. Kathy stood over us, staring down.

Me: Hey, Beautiful! I love your headband today; it's so sparkly! (brushing my hand along Doris's cheek).
Doris: (eyes popping wide open and a smile crossing her face as she strokes her head) Da boda.
Me: Doris, I need to see Mom, I'll catch up with you soon.
Doris: Da boda doonnnn…
Me: Yes, soon…

I didn't have the patience or the strength to try to understand her right then. I lightly squeezed her hand and walked to Mom's room.

Joe was already at her bedside, talking to her softly. I passed Christine's bed and noticed the silence. I placed my bag on the dresser and turned to look at Christine. I watched intensely for a moment, then started to step toward her bed.

Me: Joe?
Joe: Yea?
Me: Is Christine breathing?

I took a step closer. I was scared and looked toward Joe. His face had fallen. I gathered some strength and found myself at her side, I couldn't touch her...I placed my hand near her mouth.

Me: Honey, I don't feel any...any air moving...

I stepped back as Joe moved to the bedside. He placed his hand on Christine's neck, two fingers doing what he does, looking for a pulse. As he pulled his hand away, the aide stepped into the room. Joe looked up at her and shook his head.

Joe: (nodding toward the door, he addressed the aide) She's still warm, but she's gone.

I felt a wave of emotion come over me that I couldn't identify. My eyes burned. I looked down at my feet and turned quickly to go to Mom's side.

I sat for a moment and watched the aide pull the curtain around Christine's bed. Joe took up residency on the other side of Mom's bed. I heard whispering behind me. I looked down at Mom and a quiet sob escaped my throat. I pulled her hand to my lips.

Later in the day, Joe and I returned for our third visit of the day. I learned that Christine had fought a long fight, battles of cancer, strokes, and falls dating back to 1994. Her husband Tony was at her side the entire time. I was sorry she was gone, but happy she was at peace. I turned my attention to Mom.

It was important to make sure Mom was comfortable, it was important that I be the rock my Prince needed. I looked out the window as the rain fell, it was turning out to be Mom's favorite kind of day. I returned my gaze to Mom, she seemed comfortable, which should have brought me peace. Still, my heart hurt. Christine was a warm and special soul, she lit up when I called her name. Despite all her challenges, a smile filled her eyes when she looked at me. That was a gift I will never forget.

Rest in peace, beautiful Christine.

Angels at Every Turn

Connecticut & Florida

September 2019

My desk was piled with quotes, proposals, and contracts. A cold cup of coffee and an empty teacup sat in the corner, along with a few crumbs on a napkin from the crackers I had the night before. I had left Regency House after 8:00 p.m. and had gone straight to the studio to work. I lasted two hours before physical and emotional fatigue took its toll, I surrendered and drove home. My morning was not shaping up much better, I was exhausted, uneasy, and facing a flight back to Florida.

An internal battle had been playing out inside my head since the previous morning when I had booked the flight. On one battle hill was Mom, on the opposite hill were two client projects that needed my attention. Labor Day was behind us, which meant the holiday deliverables deadlines had passed. When I had signed on these projects the previous spring, I had assured my clients they would have a completed home upon their return to Naples over the holidays.

I have always trained my team to under promise and over deliver. I swallowed hard, was I really weighing the importance of finishing custom draperies over Mom? Who does that?

I leaned back in my chair, sipped my fresh coffee, and reflected upon my latest visit with Mom.

Me: Mom?

I gently tucked a stray hair behind her ear, her breathing was shallow yet steady. Her glasses were gone, her mouth was sunken, she no longer had her teeth, her complexion was pale but not ashen. She was almost unrecognizable.

Me: Mom? Can you hear me? Pea 2 here.

Mom took a deep breath, then resumed her steady rhythmic breathing.

Me: I gotta take a quick trip, Mom.

I swallowed hard, pushing back a hard lump that had suddenly risen in the back of my throat.

Me: I'll be back on Friday night.

Nothing, no response. She continued to sleep and breathe easy.

Me: Mom? (tears welling quickly) I don't know what to do… help me. I'm scared that if I go you won't be here when I return. I would never forgive myself if I left and you…

I couldn't finish my sentence, the tears flowed fast and heavy. Holding her hand, I laid my head on her chest and just let the tears flow. Oddly I found some comfort in the steady rise and fall of her chest.

As I laid with her, memories started flowing. I could hear her laughter fill the room, I could see her playing with Ashley and Joey and the love radiating from her bright, dancing eyes. I flashed back to countless conversations, serious and light. My mind twisted and turned, and why it went where it did, I'll never know, but a light smile crossed my face as her seventy-fifth birthday popped into my head.

Me: Do you know what today is?
MIL: No, what's today?
Me: It's your birthday, Mom!!!
MIL: Well, whadya know!?

Silence.

MIL: How old am I?
Me: Seventy-five.
MIL: What?!? No, sir! That's old!! I'm not old!
Me: (giggling) You're a spring chicken!
MIL: Chicken?
Me: Yep, a spring chicken! I love you, Mom.
MIL: I love you too, Chicken.

I laughed out loud, remembering the day vividly—Mom wearing her purple shirt with a few stains on the front from her lunch, her apple cap sitting crooked on her head, and the look of surprise that skated across her face. My emotions sharply turned as I struggled not to be angry about the loss of those precious moments.

I sat up and wiped my face with the back of my hand. I studied her face, looking for answers. I glanced at my watch, 8:05 p.m.

Me: Mom?

Nothing, just the steady breathing.

Me: Mom…I gotta go…promise me you're not going anywhere for a few days…please, Mom.

Her eyelids fluttered slightly as her eyes opened and she took a quick breath, then her lids rested easy and the rhythmic breathing resumed.

I studied her face and asked myself, was that permission or a last-ditch effort from her begging me to stay?

I pushed my chair back and shook my head. Katie was leaning against the frame of my office door.

Katie: Ready?
Me: I guess so…
Katie: You okay?
Me: I don't know…I…
Katie: Maybe you shouldn't go, maybe Darleen can take care of the measure and meet with Jay?
Me: Honestly, we're already behind on the cutoff, Cindy's workroom is making an exception to fit us in, and I can't trust Darleen will be able to do this.

I felt a wave of anger as I listened to what I was saying. I think, *What am I paying Darleen for? I shouldn't have to leave, she should be able to do this. Yet I know I can't trust that she can.* I knew that this meant I needed to address this particular problem, too. One of my most despised jobs in my career is letting employees go. I pushed the thought out of my head and picked up my bag. That was an issue I'd need to address another day. I smiled weakly at Katie and turned to leave.

Arriving in Florida after seven hours of travel, I unlocked the door to our newly leased condo. My heart was heavy. Joe had been sending me updates on Mom, saying she was mostly just sleeping and seemed comfortable. I placed my purse on the dining table and opened the slider, allowing the sound of the fountain to soothe my aching heart. The chime of my phone startled me, the screen announced Joe was calling.

Me: Hello?

Joe: Hey...

Me: You okay?

Joe: Dave's here...

Me: Joe...?

Joe: She's not doing well; I'm not sure she's going to make it through the night.

Me: How...(sucking in a quick breath, attempting to stifle a sob) I thought...I...

Joe: I don't know...

Me: Oh my God...I'm (tears breaking free)...I'm not there...how could... (choking) do this?

Joe: Honey, please...

Me: (wiping the tears that are flowing too fast) I'm going to start looking at flights for tomorrow right now.

Joe: I don't think you're going to make it.

I tried to read into his words, he had to be angry. He had to be downright pissed that I left. We'd done so much of this journey together, how could I have left him at the end? My stomach turned and I felt as if I was going to be sick. He is my rock, always there for me. Thirty years ago, he saved me from an abusive relationship and a life filled with heartache. This was my thanks to him? I could barely process what he was saying. The guilt was overwhelming.

Joe: I called the kids, told them she's close.

Me: Honey, I'm...I'm sorry.

Joe: Don't...Dave and I are going to stay...

Me: I'll let you...let you know what I find.

I disconnected the phone, looking to escape and distract myself with another task. I worked hard with an angel from God at American Express Travel who booked me on a 1:00 p.m. flight the next day out of Fort Myers, Florida, to Philadelphia, with a tight connection to Connecticut. She told me that God had a plan and if I was meant to be with Mom when she passed then I would be. I offered my thanks through my tears and looked to the heavens for strength and guidance. I placed calls to my workroom and my contractor, who transformed into angels themselves and rearranged their schedules to meet me early to accomplish a day's worth of work in three short hours.

I called Joe to share the updates, his spirits seemed a little lighter. He and Dave were spending some much needed time together, reminiscing about childhood memories and sharing stories of Mom. I imagined Mom smiling deep down, enjoying the laughter and banter between them both. Throughout the night Joe and I exchanged calls and texts every hour, keeping each other updated.

At 1:00 a.m., my phone chimed. I grabbed it on the first ring, my mind and body had not surrendered to sleep.

Joe: Hi.
Me: Hi, how is she?
Joe: Same. We've decided to go home and get a few hours of sleep.
Me: You sure?
Joe: I know this sounds crazy, but I think she's telling us to. I have this feeling of peace right now. I really don't think she's going to go yet.

For a moment my heart soared, she's going to wait for me.

Me: Okay. Try to get some rest, call me when you get up and when you get back to her please?
Joe: I will. I love you.

I pursed my lips tightly, digging for composure to be able to respond.

Me: (just above a whisper) I…I love you, too.

The phone disconnected, I laid my head back onto the pillow, still holding the phone. Sleep rushed in quickly, although it was restless. The few hours of rest were filled with dreams of Mom, she was healthy, she had a clear head, and we were our old selves.

I moved through my morning working efficiently between text updates from Joe. I arrived at the airport with my anxiety on overload, only to be met with a delay. There, behind the gate counter, God placed another angel.

Me: Hi (my voice shaking)…my name is Lisa Davenport, I'm on this flight to Philadelphia.

Gate Angel: Hi! (smiling warmly, speaking with a deep southern accent) How can I halp yooou?

Me: Well (my bottom lip quivering)...I have a tight connection, and my mother-in-law is dying. I can't miss that flight...I don't...(choking)...can I get...

Gate Angel: Oh, Darlin'...

She reached across the counter and placed a reassuring hand on top of my shaking one. Her presence offered me some temporary relief. She was present, not distracted, and clearly looking to help me.

Me: I'm in seat 32 (sniffling).

Gate Angel: Hhmmmm (lifting her reading glasses to her nose and studying the screen), let me see.

Me: If I can get just a little closer...

Gate Angel: I've got (intensely focusing on her computer)...oh, this is good! (her face lighting up like a child finding a candy jar) I can get you closer!

Me: How close (hoping against hope)?

Gate Angel: How about front row aisle?

Me: What? Yes, please! (fumbling through my purse) Here...here's my credit car...

Gate Angel: No charge (her fingers flying over the keyboard).

My eyes connected with hers, I barely kept my composure.

Me: Then...thank you.

Gate Angel: Honey, somebody is working to get you home. Your incoming flight is no longer delayed. We were waiting on the flight crew; we're all accounted for and looking at an on-time departure.

She handed me my new ticket and whispered good luck, assuring me that her prayers were with me.

I chose a seat by the window in the waiting area where I could watch the ground crews loading luggage on the plane. A small bird flew by the window and circled back, landing on a ledge at the bottom of the window. She was just inches away from where my feet are stretched; she was small, yet brave, flying and landing on an airport windowsill. She twitched, then turned her head toward me before taking flight again. I pulled out my phone, checking my text messages. There was nothing from Joe. Hoping this was good news, I dialed his number.

Joe: Hi.
Me: How we doin?
Joe: She's still here. I swear she's waiting for you.
Me: (my heart hurting) Did Ashley and Andrew make it?
Joe: Yeah, they are here, Dave and Scot, too.
Me: Good. There's an angel at the gate here, she upgraded me to the first row with my tight connection. This flight was initially delayed, but now we're taking off on time.
Joe: Good, keep me posted.
Me: I will. I love you.
Joe: Love you, too.

Angels graced my entire trip, and I needed them. Despite promising an on-time departure from Florida, my first plane sat on the tarmac for fifteen minutes. When we arrived in Philadelphia, the flight attendant held the left-side guests, allowing me to disembark first. I never shared my situation with him, how he knew, I'll never know. My connecting flight was in another terminal, which required me to engage in a full-out sprint between terminals. Travelers cleared the way without me ever saying, "Excuse me." As I approached the gate, the attendant smiled.

Gate Angel: Easy. You made it! We're fueling now and knew you were enroute.

I held my phone over the scanner and a loud beep screamed, announcing there was an issue with my ticket. Panic flowed over me. I'm a seasoned traveler, typically this wouldn't rock me.

Gate Angel: Ms. Davenport, can I see that e-ticket?

I held up my phone. She nodded and her fingers flew over the keyboard. The computer spit and coughed out a new paper ticket.

Gate Angel: Here ya go! Have a good flight.

The ticket shook slightly in my hand as I read my new seat assignment, seat 3C. I stood for a moment, studying the ticket.

Gate Angel: Everything okay, Ms. Davenport?
Me: Why the seat change?
Gate Angel: I don't know, guess it's your lucky day!

I walked down the ramp and by a window just before the jet bridge. A bird, a twin to the one in Fort Myers, sat on the sill. She turned her head toward me and took off. Watching her fly away, I texted Joe.

Text from Me: Boarding my flight…I made it and my seat is upgraded again, 3C.
Text from Joe: She's still here. Scot and Anna will pick you up.
Text from Me: Tell her I'm on my way. I just need a couple hours, tops.
Text from Joe: I will. Love you.
Text from Me: Love you, too.

The forty minutes in the air felt like a lifetime. As the tires hit the tarmac, my heart was racing. I flipped my phone from airplane mode and it sung a choir of bleeps, announcing numerous text messages. My only priority was Joe and Scot. There was nothing from Joe, my heart sunk. I texted him.

Text from Me: Landed.
Text from Joe: Good, she's still hanging on, hurry.
Text from Me: Kiss her for me, tell her I'm close.
Text from Joe: I will.

A text came in from Scot.

Text from Scot: Let us know when you land.
Text from Me: Landed.
Text from Scot: Okay, we're on our way. Meet you outside arrivals.

I paced on the sidewalk along arrivals waiting for Scot and Anna. I was uneasy, my breathing was fast and my heart was racing. I swear the young man next to me could not only hear it, but see it beating outside my chest. I texted Joe.

Text from Me: Just waiting on Scot and Anna.
Text from Joe: Okay.

Okay? I thought. I was afraid to ask why he didn't tell me Mom was still with us. Then it hit me. I saw Anna's car pulling to the curb. I slid into the back and rested my head against the seat. She was gone. I could feel it.

I didn't let on to Scot or Anna my belief, I nodded as Scot told me she was still hanging on, she had to be, Joe would have told us otherwise. We rode together—Anna updating me on the kids, me in the backseat pressing on an imaginary gas pedal trying to move the vehicle along a little faster. As we arrived at Regency House, Anna scanned the parking lot for a spot.

Anna: I'll need to go around again.
Me: Can you drop me at the door?
Anna: Of course.

I bolted into the lobby, running past the receptionist without signing in. She didn't stop me, I wondered if she knew. My hands shook almost uncontrollably as I punched the code into the keypad to gain access to Mom's unit. As I stepped through the doors, Katy, Mom's nurse, was standing at her rolling computer in the middle of the hallway.

Me: Katy…Katy…did I make it?!?

Katy closed her eyes and shook her head no.

Me: No…No…noooo…

I burst beyond her and pushed open the door to Mom's room. The room was quiet, Joe started to cross the room toward me, opening his arms.

Me: No, Mom…no (shaking my head, tears running so quickly down my checks that they drip off my chin).

I tossed my purse on Christine's old bed and fell onto Mom's bed, sobbing uncontrollably, begging for forgiveness for not being with her. Her body was cool as I rested my palm on her cheek and struggled to catch my breath. A strong hand squeezed my shoulder, I didn't need to turn to see who was there to offer me comfort. I know his touch; I could feel his energy radiating through me. Failure washed over me. I had failed Joe, Mom, and the kids. I had mistakenly thought I had enough time. How would they ever forgive me?

Joe guided me into a sitting position, then helped me stand. He wrapped me in his arms and held me tight as we released eight years of stress through tears. I turned and saw Scot and Anna in the doorway. I waved toward the bed, offering them their own time.

Ashley, Joey, and Andrew materialized before my eyes. I had been so focused on Mom that I never noticed they were in the room. Their arms encircled me. We held each other, tears flowed, and comfort seeped through our souls.

Katy gently pushed the door open and approached myself and Joe.

Katy: I'm going to need a little time with your Mom. The funeral home will be here shortly.
Joe: Yes of course, can they say their last goodbyes?
Katy: Of course.

Joe instructed the family that we would need to clear the room shortly to allow Katy to do her job. I scanned the room. Mom would have been proud. The room was filled with those who loved her. I knew she had enjoyed the time that Dave and Joe shared the previous night. That morning, Scot and Joe bantered in their own way.

As we cleared the room for Katy, she invited us to stay after she was done until the funeral director arrived.

Katy finished, waved the family back into Mom's room, and approached Joe and me.

Katy: She's all set and ready to go. You'll see I opened the window…to let her spirit fly.
Me: Thank you for everything, Katy.
Katy: (caressing my arm) I couldn't let her go until you got here.

Behind her eyeglasses the tears gathered in her eyes.

Katy: She loved you so much. She waited for you, you just weren't meant to see her go.

I hugged Katy tight, another angel sent to me that night. As I pushed the door to Mom's room open, I noticed the atmosphere had changed slightly. While it wasn't joyful, it was definitely a little lighter. I lifted my chin as the tears flowed again. *You did good, Mom.* I thought. *You're free now to start your next chapter.*

Outside the window, a bird, a triplet to the two that joined me earlier that day, sat on the bird feeder. I studied her closely. She jumped onto the roof of the birdhouse, turned her head toward the window, and took flight. She flew around the gazebo and back by the window before disappearing into the setting sun.

Safe travels and God speed, Beautiful. You're free! I love you and miss you already.

Later that night, over a glass of wine and a pile of balled up tissues, I learned how Mom's last moments unfolded. Around the time I was taking off out of Philadelphia, Dave and Scot left Mom's room, Dave to go home for a bit, Scot to do the same and pick me up. Joe encouraged Ashley and Andrew to take a break themselves. They refused. Ashley felt a tug, and she listened.

Mom took her last breath just a few short moments after Joe kissed her and told her I was close, that I had landed safely.

She wasn't alone. Joe wasn't alone. They had two angels at their sides—Ashley and Andrew.

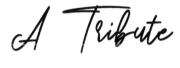

A Tribute

Connecticut

September 2019

The house is so quiet. Upstairs the kids sleep deeply, as they should; broken hearts often bring a deep sleep. Joe and I, despite our own broken hearts, were up before the sun with an emptiness we couldn't quite understand.

Joe: (reaching across the sofa caressing my leg) Honey?
Me: Yeah?
Joe: I want you to write the obituary.
Me: Me? Will your family be okay with that?

He looked down into his coffee cup and nodded his head. As if I didn't have enough emotions running on overload; this request put me over the edge. My already swollen eyes welled up with tears again.

Me: I don't know…I'm not sure I can…(my voice breaking) find the right words.
Joe: (squeezing my leg gently) My Mom (a tear escaping his bloodshot eyes)… my Mom wouldn't want a traditional obituary. Years ago, she told you to tell her story…your story. Think of it as the final chapter.

I closed my eyes as a sob broke away from the back of my throat. I was honored that he felt I was the right person to tell the world about Mom. I worried, though, that I wouldn't find the words and, most of all, I was concerned about how the idea of me writing Mom's obituary would be received from the rest of Joe's family.

Joe handed me my laptop and kissed my forehead.

This is Mom's obituary, as I wrote it, and as it appeared in the *Middletown Press* (Middletown, Connecticut) and the *Carroll County News* (Berryville, Arkansas).

Rosemary Zieroth, Durham, CT, passed away Friday, September 6, 2019, at the Regency House in Wallingford.

Somewhere, on the other side, there is a leather recliner, the Sunday *NY Times* crossword puzzle, and a steaming cup of coffee sitting in front of a large picture window filled with plants, blue glass, and crystals. Of course, it is a perfect day, the rain gently and rhythmically dances down the glass while a light, cool breeze passes over the top of the newspaper, lifting just the edge.

An amazing woman has taken up residency here, she is free of all pain, confusion, and despair.

She sits and smiles widely as the view is now crystal clear as she watches her beloved children. Her eldest, innovative and clever Cynthia Fisk with her husband Scottie and her son Cody. Then her first son, the resourceful John Davenport, his wife Linda and their three boys Rory, Marc, and Shane. She throws her head back in a fit of laughter as she watches her forever comedian, joker, and talented son David with his beautiful wife Violet and their children Christopher and Timmy. She folds the paper and shakes her head lovingly as she watches her bright, "favorite son" Scot with his graceful wife Anna and their children Theo and Sophia. Then she leans back and proudly folds her arms across her chest as she watches her compassionate, insightful baby boy, her caretaker and fierce advocate, Joe with his lovely wife Lisa and their children Ashley and Joey. She lifts her chin with great satisfaction and nods, knowing she did well.

She sips her coffee as she watches her companion for the last several years and gives him a nod of thanks for the good times. She stretches her legs, crossing them at the ankles and watches the movie of her life. It is filled with great memories of her home, often filled with those in need, of road trips halfway across the country to see her children and grandchildren. It is abundant with accomplishments. She was a fierce advocate for women, amazing poet, writer, and wordsmith. An editor, a technical writer and amateur photographer.

She rises easy out of the recliner, stretches, and turns her head toward the sound of her dad's blacksmith shop in the distance. She places a large floppy hat upon her head and tips it toward the direction of all her beloved and silently reminds them all she is forever with them. As her skirt spins, she heads down the hill to join her sisters, Grace and Frieda, with a little skip in her step.

The family would like to send a special message of gratitude and love to the angels at Regency House Star Unit for their compassion, love, and unwavering dedication to Rosemary's care.

In lieu of flowers, donations are requested for Alzheimer's Association (https://alz.org).

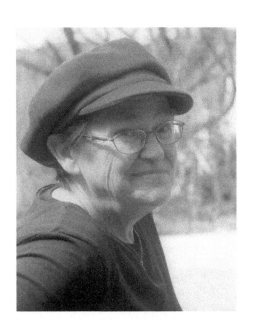

Epilogue: Summer 2020

Florida

The TSA line isn't overly long or crowded. An agent barked orders behind her mask, I studied her for a moment, thinking *How does she not have a ripping headache from trying to project her voice through that mask?* My right shoulder began to ache from the weight of my black bag. I shifted my weight from my right hip to my left, hoping to disperse the weight as I watched less-seasoned travelers attempt to navigate the screening process.

A tall, very distinguished man with a thick Jamaican accent is attempting to follow the directions through the muffled mask. He was obviously confused as he leaned in closer to try and understand.

TSA agent: Fauuud, in a seportate ban. Seporate aut aloctronics lurger thun your cell phane. Shows. All in a ban! Camputars in a seportate ban!

I quickly translated the muffled directions, "In bins, food, shoes, electronics larger than your cell phone and computers in a separate bin."

Distinguished gentleman: My shoes in separate container?
TSA agent: No sir! Camputars in a seportate ban!
 Distinguished gentleman: (in an ever so proper fashion) My apologies, kind
    lady, but my shoes and my food in a separate container, correct?
TSA agent: Dew you have a camputar?!
Distinguished gentleman: No, but I have a tablet…

TSA agent: Walllll, thut is aloctronics lurger thun your cell phane. Seportate ban!

I watched the distinguished gentleman carefully as he slowly calculated his next steps. He placed shoes and tablet into one bin and his prepackaged sandwich into another. His eyes darted left to right as he examined the bins, at the last second, he pulled his tablet out of the bin and added it to the bin with his sandwich. He stood tall, looking accomplished.

TSA: Sarrr! Seportate bans!

I pulled my laptop out of my bin and slid it to my newfound friend.

Me: Sir? Here, drop your tablet in here.
Distinguished gentleman: Separated container?
Me: Today, yes. These rules change daily!
Distinguished gentleman: (a cloud falling over his eyes) Thank you for helping me.
Me: My pleasure.

I turned to pick up another empty bin. I placed my computer in the bin and closed the zipper of my black travel bag. As I do, I see the edge of a purple binder, the binder holds years of memories of my life with MIL. She told me years ago, to tell her story. "It may be the only way for me to help others," she had said. *Mom,* I thought. *You've taught me so much, thank you. It's time to share your story.*

About the Author

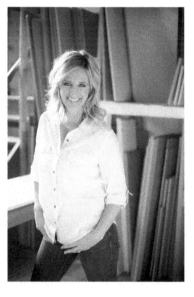

Lisa Davenport has been telling stories through fine custom interiors and exteriors for more than twenty-five years. After all, great designs tell a story.

In 2012, while her mother-in-law was slipping away from her into the depths of Alzheimer's, Lisa started sharing their journey as random Facebook posts. She never expected those short little stories would be so well received. So well, in fact, that numerous followers and friends, including her mother-in-law, encouraged her to write a book. As a dyslexic, Lisa was crippled by fear when it came to writing. How could she write an entire book? Believing it truly does take a village, Lisa surrounded herself with those who could guide her through the process while still preserving her own signature on the design of this very important story.

Lisa splits her time between her hometown of Durham, Connecticut, where her roots run deep, and Naples, Florida, where she has welcomed and embraced by a new group of "family" and friends. While she loves sharing her own little "Mayberry" (aka Durham) with her clients and followers, she is also smitten with the charm of Naples.

Lisa is an active member in both her communities. In Connecticut she is a long-serving member of the Durham Fair Association assisting her husband, Joe. In Florida she serves as an advisory board member of Valerie's House, a special place for children and families to connect to heal after experiencing the death of a loved one. Lisa has also dedicated much of her time to missionary work in the eastern mountains of Kentucky, granting her the distinction of being named a Kentucky Colonel by Governor Steve Bashear.

Lisa is married to the love of her life, Joe, and she can't imagine this ride called life without him. Together they have two children, Ashley and Joey. In 2021, they welcomed their new grandson, Flynn, into their hearts and lives.

A portion of the proceeds from *Life with MIL* will be donated to the Alzheimer's Association.